Easy Method of ACUPUNCTURE

Based on
Meridian Theory

WATANABE Hiroshi M.D.Ph.D.

PREFACE

In 1972, news of acupuncture anesthesia was widely reported in newspapers, causing a worldwide sensation as an unbelievable story. This news strongly impressed me too, and made me interested in acupuncture. By chance, a colleague of mine had an opportunity to visit the Department of Anesthesiology of Tokyo Medical-&-Dental University and observe acupuncture treatment. We tried to apply acupuncture therapy by "the Tokyo Medical-&-Dental University's method" on patients complaining lumber pain and asking for acupuncture therapy. We were quite astonished by and satisfied of the excellent effects. There I started studying acupuncture seriously. It was in April 1973.

Yet after reading many books, attending lectures, and observing acupuncture treatment by many professional acupuncturists, I was further impressed by the diversity in the principles and technical methods practiced by different acupuncturist. The enormous amount of the names and functions of acupuncture points etc. were also a surprise. Indeed, the barrier between the concept and terms of acupuncture world and those of Occidental Medicine is revealed to be more solid and higher than expected. Some may look Five Element Theory suspicious or superstitious. Perhaps, it is cleverer to take the acupuncture world as a new field or a different world for human body function. So I tried to establish more simplified system by modifying the Tokyo Medical-&-Dental University method based on the Meridian Theory, probably based on the method of the late Dr. NAGAYAMA Kunzou.

The method of Tokyo Medical-&-Dental University which we understood is as mentioned below.
1. Meridian selection: Those passing through the location of complaints.
2. Point selection: On the meridian, distal from elbow-or-knee joint, bilaterally.
3. Needle insertion: Vertical.
4. Stimulation: 45Hz cathode rectangular electric stimulation.
    As strong as the patient can endure.
    Strength of each point is to be felt equal.

Today, this method is largely modified through experiences. But the fundamental conditions such as the meridian-&-point selection and balance taking stimulation are still in the same way.

Hereinafter the system described here was established by myself. The characteristics of this system are as described below.

1. The system is completely due to Meridian Theory.

    Fundamental meridian selection is to select the meridian that passes through the location of complaint or the meridian that has close relation with corresponding ORGAN (in the meaning of Oriental Medicine). Thereby the meridians of classic literature are considered important, and relation of similarity between ORGAN and anatomical organ bearing other name (such as KIDNEY and adrenal body) or special ideas of Oriental Medicine (such as the relation between LUNG and skin & hair) is taken into consideration.

   This method does not require difficult dialectics or consideration of "ORGAN Diagnosis" under complicated diagnosis of Oriental Medicine.
2. Meridians to be treated are selected at the beginning of the treatment according to the above mentioned principle, being different from generally adopted method in other schools.
3. Points are selected on above mentioned meridian, without consideration of "function of the point" which is described minutely in other textbooks.
   Principally "local point locating" is not adopted.
4. Points are taken principally at periphery of extremities, i.e. distal from elbow and knee joint, bilaterally.
5. Basic method of treatment is electro-acupuncture. Supplementation-&-Draining is performed according to the oral teaching of the late Dr. MANAKA Yoshio.
   Stimulation is controlled so as the patient feels the stimulation comfortable and equal at all points.
6. Retaining needle, moxa needle, intradermal needle, thumbtack needle and acupoint injection are performed under the completely same principle as electro-acupuncture.
7. In acupoint injection, injection is used mainly as stimulation, without expecting pharmacological effects. So, in most cases any substances for subcutaneous-or-intramuscular use can be used. This method is useful also as an entrance of acupuncture. When pharmacologically active substances are used, the effects are much stronger with less dose, and it continues much longer.

   These principles of acupuncture treatment are (often widely) different from usually adopted ones. They may look easygoing methods. However, excellent effects are obtained for many symptoms and diseases by the treatment under these principles as mentioned later.

   This method has no side effect except slight pain of needle insertion and bruise due to subcutaneous bleeding. Other "side effects" such as infection, needle breakage or burn by moxa needle are completely avoidable by normal attention.

   There are numerous indications of acupuncture. In textbooks or clinical reports, many points and methods for many diseases are described. But, in this book, only my experiences with sure results are described.

   I believe that this method is one of the easiest methods of acupuncture. Especially Acupoint Injection of my style can be used by medical doctors, dentists and nurses who have almost no knowledge of acupuncture under the same principle.

HOW TO USE THIS BOOK

This book is written mainly for the medical doctors and dentists who have no experiences in acupuncture up to the present. As acupuncture is a method of Oriental Medicine, principles and using instruments are quite unfamiliar ones from those used in Occidental Medicine.

The approach of the system of acupuncture described in this book is almost absolutely based on the Meridian Theory, and it is a very simple system established by myself. It will encourage beginners to learn acupuncture practice.

A number of same words are used both in Oriental Medicine and in Occidental Medicine that have quite different meanings. For example, water in Occidental Medicine is H_2O, whereas in Oriental Medicine it is colorless fluid circulating in the body, like lymph fluid, extracellular fluid or intracellular fluid etc. To avoid confusion, words used in Oriental Medicine are written in capitals like WATER in this book.

The use of this book will be more efficient by following the orders given below.

[1st] To Comprehend Meridians and the Outline of Meridians' Routes

The present method is based on the Meridian Theory. So, it is very important to understand meridians and their routes. For this purpose, read Part 1 (OUTLINE OF ACUPUNCTURE) carefully with the following comments in mind.

① Go through briefly PART1, Chapter 1 §1 & §2 and Chapter 2, leaving §2 (p.5) and Chapter 3 (p.9~11).

② Read carefully PART I Chapter 4 §1 to 3 (Meridian and Acupuncture point, p.12~43). Chapter 4 may be one of the most incomprehensive part of this book. But, in this step, there is no need to make effort to remember details. It is enough to read the descriptions of individual meridian in the frame seeing meridian chart (or meridian doll, if possible) and to get overall idea of the meridian routes. There are some differences in the routes among different charts. But there is no need to mind minute differences of charts. In this step, the main purpose of Chapter 4 is to understand and to get rough idea about the meridians and points. Here, at least, the names of meridians such as "LUNG Meridian" etc. and the outline of their routes are to be remembered.

③ Go through descriptions PART1 Chapter 4 §4 [1] and [2] (p.44~46). Description [3] (names and locations of acupuncture points p.46~63) should be regarded as a telephone book. This part can be used not only for the affirmation of the location of points but also for the reconfirmation of the routes and local distribution & their flow direction. This troublesome work will be good help for understanding meridians and acupuncture points very much.

[2nd] To Understand Diagnosis for Acupuncture (Part2 Chapter 3 & 4, p.70~79)

Medical examination for acupuncture is quite different from that of Occidental Medicine. Here questioning and pulse diagnosis are the most important.

To understand the questioning, it is necessary to read PART2 Chapter 1 §3 (Questioning p.66) and PART4 Chapter 1 §3 (106~107) carefully.

In PART2 (Medical Examination for Acupuncture), Chapter 1 §1, 2, 4 (p.64~67) can be run over lightly. But much more effort must be given to read Chapter 2 (p.68 ~69) and Chapter3 and Chapter 4 (p.70~79).

For the pulse diagnosis, it is important to read the description of PART2 Chapter3 carefully. That is:
1. To remember the location of "Sunkou$^{(Jp.)}$ (or "Sun$^{(Jp.)}$" or Front Position), "Kanjou$^{(Jp.)}$" (or "Kan$^{(Jp.)}$" or Middle Position) and "Shakuchuu$^{(Jp.)}$" (or "Shaku$^{(Jp.)}$" or Rear Position).
2. To understand the pulse of "Fu$^{(Jp.)}$" (Float) and "Chin$^{(Jp.)}$" (Sink), and to practice the method of examination of "Fu" and "Chin".
3. To master the relations between Sun/Kan/Shaku-&-Fu/Chin$^{(Jp.)}$ and 12 Meridians.

Methods of pulse diagnosis are mentioned in PART2 Chapter3 (p70~74) in detail.

[3rd] To read through PART2 Chapter 4 (Meridian Selection), Chapter 5 (Point Selection) and Chapter 6 (Point Search) (p.75~85)

This part is very important only in practicing acupuncture therapy. So in the first step, there is no need to read this part too seriously. Read those again carefully when you start acupuncture therapy.

[4th] To Practice "Puncture with Fine Needle"

Before the start of practicing, it is necessary to read PART3 Chapter 1 §2 (Management of Filiform Needle (p.89~93) carefully.
1. It is recommended to start training on soft test bench.
2. Read PART3 §2 [3] and [4] (p.89~93) carefully, and practice puncture following to the directions given in [4] D (Training of Skin Cutting and Needle Penetration, p.93)
3. Before applying acupuncture on the patient, it is necessary to read again §2 (management of filiform needle, p.89~93) carefully, and understand the descriptions well.

[5th] To Understand the Method of Supplementation and Draining

For this purpose, it will be useful to read this book in following order.
① Read again PART2 Chapter2 (Deficiency-&-Excess and Supplementation -&-Draining p.68~69)
② Read again PART3 Chapter 2 §1 (Management of Needle and Supplementation -&-Draining, (97~98) and §2 (method of stimulation and Supplementation -&-Draining p.98~103) carefully.

③ Read carefully PART3 §2 [5] (Electro-acupuncture p.103), then read PART4 Chapter 2 §2 (Electro-acupuncture109~115), especially [2] (Instrument for Electric Stimulation111~115) carefully.

[6th] **To Confirm Understanding about Meridians, Meridian Selection and Point Selection**

It is useful to read again PART2 Chapter 4, 5, 6 (p.75~85) carefully for this purpose.

Thus the lecture of basic outline about the system of my method of acupuncture is completed. Read again Part 4 and Part5, and try to practice acupuncture referring to PART6.

It is important to pay enough attention to next 3 points.
1. Faultless disinfection is necessary not to cause infection.
2. When a needle is bent, change the needle immediately to avoid needle breakage.
3. Careful attention must be paid to avoid burn by moxa needle.

Except these three possible accidents, there is no risk in this method of acupuncture. The best way to become proficient in acupuncture is to practice. Ideal objects of acupuncture for beginners are pain, shoulder stiffness, pollinosis, dysmenorrhea and attack of bronchial asthma. They are easy to make a plan of treatment, and the effects appear quickly and clearly.

Some doctors may vaguely feel opposition to acupuncture. For such cases, it is recommended to begin with acupoint injection.

The world of acupuncture is multiple. This method is only a small part of acupuncture. Those who have enough experiences of acupuncture will feel incongruous with this description. But methods of acupuncture may be (or should be) essentially diverse, and any method is valuable as far as it is effective.

The easiest acupuncture

Probably, there are many doctors who want mainly (or only) to get prompt results of acupuncture, not expecting to be a specialist of acupuncture. For this purpose, there is an excellent and very easy method.

That is ACUPOINT INJECTION.

Acupuncture is a therapeutic method to insert needles to some points (acupoints) and to give some stimulation.

Theoretically any kind of needle and any kind of stimulation can be used as acupuncture. When the needle is switched from acupuncture needle to injection needle, and stimulation from electricity to injection, that is namely my method of acupoint injection. Acupoint injection involves more pain than usual acupuncture, and causes bruise more frequently. But it is much easier to practice than any method of acupuncture. It does not demand paying consideration to Deficiency-or-Excess of meridians nor exact hitting on acupoint. I believe that this is the easiest introduction to acupuncture.

For this purpose, please use this book as mentioned below:
1. Read "Acupoint Injection" (PART4 Chapter 3 §5, p.121 ~ 122) over and over until you understand well. (That may not be difficult for doctors.)
2. Use "Frequently Used Points and Their Location" (PART1 Chapter 4 [3] B p.46 ~ 63) and "Practice of Acupuncture" (PART6, p.134 ~ 219) as "telephone directory". The direction of needle puncture is vertical to the skin.

The late Dr. MANAKA published an introduction book named "The Layman's Guide to Acupuncture". Acupoint injection may be also suitably called "The Layman's Practical Acupuncture".

Anyway, at your start of present purpose, there is no need to read other parts of this book **NOW**.

However, it is strongly recommended:
1. To confirm every time the location of aimed point by "Frequently Used Points and Their Location" (PART I Chapter 4 [3] B (p.48 ~ 63). Frequently used points are written in bold letters.
2. To habituate to stroke softly around the aimed point before injection. This habit will help you to get tactile sense of acupoint so much.
3. In PART 6 , there may be found many matters which you hardly understand. You had better not to avoid the troublesome work to seek their explanation in this book as far as you have time.

When you get skillful with this method with good effects, and yet you get interest in acupuncture, please read this book again. Thereby, it will be the best way to read in the next order. That is:

① "My Method of Meridian selection" (PART2 Chapter4 §1(p.75 ~ 79).
② "Methods of Point Search" (PART2 Chapter6 (p.83 ~ 85)

Then, you will gradually understand the meaning of my method. If you have still interest in acupuncture, please read this book again in the recommended order of "How to Use This Book". It will lead you to a new world of acupuncture.

EXPLANATORY NOTES

§ 1. Meridian

Many kinds of atlas of meridian (including meridian doll) are generally available. There, all the meridians are illustrated on the skin like a road map of a guide book. Their descriptions are not always equal, and there is no "standardized road map of meridian" yet. Hereafter atlas of this type is called "general (meridian) chart" in this book.

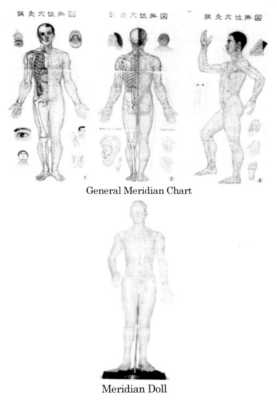

General Meridian Chart

Meridian Doll

Fig1.　Meridian Chart and Meridian Doll

Description in the general charts is quite different from that in the classic literatures. The greatest difference is in the branch of meridian. In the general charts, no branch of meridians in classic literature is described except STOMACH- and BLADDER- Meridian. In general charts, some branch of classic literature is shown as a main route of the meridian (chief meridian), and a part (sometimes almost all) of the original trunk is omitted. Some of these omitted meridians or branches are often very important for acupuncture therapy. Those routes are described as far as possible. In classc literatures, there is no atlas of meridians like general charts, and sometimes the route of meridian is described without figures. So, the route of classic literature is called "route of classic literature" or "classic meridian" in this book.

In this book, the meridians of classic literatures are principally described according to the description of the original text of Reisuu[1)(Jp.)] (霊枢 Yellow Emperor's Inner Classic, Spiritual Axis) and partly of Somon[2)(Jp.)] (素問 Yellow Emperor's Inner Classic, Simple Question). When the pathway is not clear, references are made to the diagrams of SAWADA Ken[3)] (hereafter this diagram is referred to "SAWADA's chart).

When the description among SAWADA's chart, general chart and the authors' view are different, the differences are described at the end of description of the course of each meridian (in bracket, in small letters) for reference.

§ 2. Names and Illustration of "ORGANs" (ZOU-FU[(Jp)])

"ORGAN" is called "ZOU-FU" in Oriental Medicine. However the concept of "ZOU-FU" is different from that of "organ" of Occidental Medicine. "ZOU-FU" means not only the morphological ORGAN itself, but also the function of the ORGAN. Some ZOU-FU bears the same name of the Occidental organ. But the two, for example "SPLEEN" and spleen, are to be regarded to have different meanings as if they bear the same name. It may be illogical to illustrate ZOU-FU with organs of anatomically same name.

In this book, names of ZOU-FU are written by using capital letters as "LUNG", and they are illustrated with circle, at the center of the body (except LUNG and KIDNEY which are illustrated at both side of the body) independent of the location of organs of anatomically same name.

§ 3. Illustration of Meridians

Single meridian is shown as solid line, chief meridian as thick solid line, and branches as fine line. The direction of its flow is shown with arrow marks. The main branch of STOMACH meridian that goes down from ST_5 to ST_{45} is shown in medium thick line. The course to ZOU-FU is illustrated schematically simplified because it is unknown. Meridians that should pass through deep parts of the body are shown in dotted lines. When both the figures of classic chart and those of general chart are shown in pair, the classic figure is shown on the left half of the body, and that of general chart on the right half of the body.

When pleural meridians are illustrated, each is printed in different color, principally according to the colors of "the FIVE ELEMENT Theory". The meridian of METAL (LU & LI), whose color is white, is shown in brown. GOVERNOR VESSEL and CONCEPTION VESSEL are shown in green line. There are two pairs of meridians of FIRE (HT-SI and PC-TE). The former, HT and SI, are colored in pink, and the latter,

PC and TE, in orange. Yo-u$^{(Jp.)}$(Yang$^{(Chn.)}$) meridians are shown in dark color, and In$^{(Jp.)}$ (Yin$^{(Ch.)}$) meridians are shown in light color, and Deep parts are illustrated in dotted lines.

The routes of general chart are illustrated on the right half of the body, and that of classic meridian, including their branches, are illustrated on the left half of the body.

§ 4. Location of Acupuncture Points

Principle of point selection is different in each school. Generally, points are selected around the location of complaints, at chest, at abdomen or at back etc. Whereas in my method, these points are seldom selected but points at peripheral parts of extremities (distal from elbow-and-knee joints) are mainly selected. In this book, frequently used points in my method are mainly described.

(Points seem to locate not always at the same fixed position. It may be quite reasonable that locations of points in every chart are often different, and it seems to me there is no exact fixed point which can be fit for everybody. So, in my opinion, points of charts should be regarded to be rough standard.)

§ 5. Code Names & Spelling of Meridians and Points

Code names of meridians and the points are given according to the code name book of WHO (STANDARD ACUPUNCTURE NOMENCLATURE[5]). In this code name book, Chinese names are also given in modern Chinese letters and modern Chinese spelling in Roman letters (Ping-in). In this book, mostly WHO Code Name is used.

Widely used Chinese-originated names such as LU$_1$ (Chung-Fu$^{(Eng.)}$, Tchong-fou$^{(Fr.)}$ etc.) are not convenient to remember.

Each Chinese letter has its meaning(s). In the Chinese-letter-using world, the meaning of the points can be understood easily. But in other area, names written in Chinese letters have no meaning, and the learners of acupuncture are forced to memorize the meaningless names of points. It may be a stressful hard work.

It seems better to remember translated English name. But it is sometimes very difficult to tell the correct nuance of the Oriental meaning of the words. For example, for the proper explanation of the word 陰 In$^{(Jp.)}$・Yin$^{(Ch.)}$ and 陽 YO-U$^{(Jp.)}$・YANG$^{(Ch.)}$, it would require several pages of explanation. Translation of 三陰交 SP$_6$ (Crossroad of 3 Yin) is quite correct, but that of 然谷 KI$_2$ (Blazing valley) is completely different (that means "Valley of the Navicular Bone").

In this book, as names of acupuncture points, WHO Code Name is mainly used. In PART1 Chapter4 §4, four types of names of points, namely WHO Code Name, traditional (not simplified) Chinese letters (Han-Zu$^{(Ch.)}$, Kanji$^{(Jp.)}$), English name and translated English name are listed. In other parts, only WHO Code Name is used.

§ 6. Personal Names

In this book, personal names are mentioned according to the order of the native land of the person. To avoid confusion, family name is written all in capital letters.

§ 7. Name of Oriental Medicine

In Japan, Oriental Medicine (≠ traditional Chinese medicine, because it is transformed and systematized into a specific system in Japan) is called "Kampo$^{(Jp.)}$". Kampo Medicine includes treatment with herbal formulas and with acupuncture. Treatment with medicine is more commonly used than acupuncture among the Japanese medical doctors. So, in this book, "Kampo" refers to the treatment with herbal formulas.

§ 8. Abbreviations

1. ORGAN and Meridian

ORGAN	Abbreviation	Meridian	Abbreviation
LUNG	LU	LUNG Meridian	LU (Merid.)
LARGE INTESTINE	LI	LARGE INTESTINE Meridian	LI (Merid.)
STOMACH	ST	STOMACH Meridian	ST (Merid.)
SPLEEN	SP	SPLEEN Meridian	SP (Merid.)
HEART	HT	HEART Meridian	HT (Merid.)
SMALL INTESTINE	SI	SMALL INTESTINE Meridian	SI (Merid.)
BLADDER	BL	BLADDER Meridian	BL (Merid.)
KIDNEY	KI	KIDNEY Meridian	KI (Merid.)
PERICARDIUM	PC	PERICARDIUM Meridian	PC (Merid.)
TRIPLE ENERGIZER	TE	TRIPLE ENERGIZER Meridian	TE (Merid.)
UPPER ENERGIZER	UE	GALLBLADDER MERIDIAN	GB (Merid.)
MIDDLE ENERGIZER	ME	LIVER Meridian	LR (Merid.)
LOWER ENERGIZER	LE	GOVERNOR VESSEL	GV
GALLBLADDER	GB	CONCEPTION Vessel	CV
LIVER	LR		

2. Symbol

Word	Abbreviation
More than	↑
Excess	⇑
Less than	↓
Defficient	⇓

3 Others

Word	Abbreviation
Finger-breadth	fb.
Meridian	Merid.
Acupuncture	acp.
Chinese	(Ch.)
English	(Eng.)
French	(Fr.)
Japanese	(Jp.)
Bone Proportional Cun	B-cun

CONTENTS

	Page
HOW TO USE THIS BOOK	iii
The easiest acupuncture	v
EXPLANATORY NOTES	vii
CONTENTS	xii

PART 1　INTRODUCTION — OUTLINE OF ACUPUNCTURE — ··· (1)

  Chapter 1　Principle and Characteristics of Acupuncture ··· (1)
    § 1 Principle of Acupuncture ··· 1
    § 2 Merits and Demerits of Acupuncture ··· 2
      [1] Merits of Acupuncture ··· 2
      [2] Demerits of Acupuncture ··· 3

  Chapter 2　Indications and Methods of Acupuncture ··· (5)
    § 1 Indications of Acupuncture ··· 5
    § 2 Methods of Acupuncture ··· 5
      [1] Principles of Acupuncture Therapy ··· 6
      [2] Methods of Stimulation ··· 6
      [3] Acupuncture without Acupuncture Needle ··· 7

  Chapter 3　Acupuncture Needles ··· (9)
    § 1 Filiform Needle(毫鍼 Goushin) ··· 9
    § 2 Intradermal Needle (in Narrow Sense) ··· 10
    § 3 Thumbtack Type Needle (En-pishin) (Thumbtack Needle) ··· 11

  Chapter 4　Meridian and Acupuncture Point ··· (12)
    § 1 Meridian & Acupuncture Point (Acupoint or Point) ··· 12
    § 2 Flow of KI(QI) and Ketsu(BLOOD) in the Meridian ··· 14
    § 3 Fourteen Meridians and Acupuncture Therapy ··· 15
      [1] LUNG Meridian(LU) ··· 15
      [2] LARGE INTESTINE Meridian (LI) ··· 17
      [3] STOMACH Meridian (ST) ··· 18
      [4] SPLEEN Meridian (SP) ··· 20
      [5] HEART Meridian (HT) ··· 22
      [6] SMALL INTESTINE Meridian ··· 24
      [7] BLADDER Meridian (BL) ··· 25
      [8] KIDNEY Meridian (KI) ··· 28
      [9] PERICARDIUM Meridian (PC) ··· 31
      [10] TRIPLE ENERGIZER Meridian (TE) ··· 32
      [11] GALLBLADDER Meridian (GB) ··· 34
      [12] LIVER Meridian (LR) ··· 37
      [13] GOVERNOR VESSEL (GV) ··· 39

[14] CONCEPTION VESSEL (CV) ··· 41
[15] Important Meridians That are not Described in Usual Charts ······ 42
§ 4 Acupuncture Point (Acupoint) ·· 44
[1] What is Acupuncture Point? ··· 44
[2] Name of Points and Their Notation ···································· 45
[3] Frequently Used Points and Their Location ·························· 46
  A. Bone Proportional Cun(abbreviation B-cun) (尺度法 Shakudohou) ···· 46
  B. Points of Each Meridian ·· 47
    1 Points of LUNG Meridian (LU) ····································· 48
    2 Points of LARGE INTESTINE Meridian (LI) ······················ 49
    3 Points of STOMACH Meridian (ST) ································ 51
    4 Points of SPLEEN Meridian (SP) ··································· 52
    5 Points of HEART Meridian (HT) ··································· 53
    6 Points of SMALL INTESTINE Meridian (SI) ······················ 54
    7 Points of Bladder Meridian (BL) ··································· 55
    8 Points of KIDNEY Meridian (KI) ··································· 56
    9 Points of PERICARDIUM Meridian (PC) ·························· 58
    10 Points of TRIPLE ENERGIZER Meridian (TE) ·················· 59
    11 Points of GALLBLADDER Meridian (GB) ························ 60
    12 Points of LIVER Meridian (LR) ··································· 61
    13 Points of GOVERNOR VESSEL (GV) ······························ 62
    14 Points of CONCEPTION VESSEL ··································· 63

PART 2　MEDICAL EXAMINATION FOR ACUPUNCTURE ················ (64)
  Chapter 1 Medical Examination of Oriental Medicine ···················· (64)
    § 1 Diagnosis by Observation ··· 65
    § 2 Diagnosis by Hearing & Smelling ···································· 65
    § 3 Diagnosis by Questioning ··· 66
    § 4 Diagnosis by Palpation ·· 66
    [1] Palpation of Abdomen ·· 66
    [2] Palpation of Meridians ··· 67
    [3] Pulse Diagnosis ·· 67
  Chapter 2 Deficiency & Excess and Supplementation & Draining ······ (68)
  Chapter 3 Pulse Diagnosis ·· (70)
    § 1 Method of Pulse Taking ·· 72
    [1] Condition of Patient ·· 72
    [2] Posture of Patient and Position of Examiner ···················· 72
    § 2 Method of Pulse Examination ······································· 72
    § 3 Judgment and Recording of Pulse ·································· 73
    [1] Estimation of Pulse ··· 73
    [2] Recording of Pulse ·· 73
  Chapter 4 Meridian Selection ·· (75)

§ 1 My Method of Meridian Selection ························· 75
§ 2 Meridian Selection According to the Location of Complaints ············ 75
§ 3 Meridian Selection according to the Relation
between ORGAN and Organ &/or Tissue ················ 76
§ 4 Meridian Selection According to the Resemblance
between ORGAN and organ in Different Name ············ 77
§ 5 Meridian Selection according to FIVE ELEMENTS Theory ············ 78
Chapter 5 Point Selection ························· (80)
§ 1 Strategy of Point Selection ························· 80
§ 2 Points at Auricle ························· 81
§ 3 HIRATA's Twelve Reaction Zone ························· 81
Chapter 6 Methods of Point Search ························· (83)
§ 1 Bone Proportional CUN (B-CUN) (Shakudohou) ············ 83
§ 2 Point Search by Electric Resistance of the Skin ············ 83
§ 3 Point Search by Palpation or Inspection ················ 84
§ 4 Point Search by Tenderness for Pressure or Puncture Pain ············ 85

PART 3 MANAGEMENT OF NEEDLE AND
STIMULATION & SUPPLEMENTATION-DRAINING ············ (86)

Chapter 1 Management of Needle ························· (86)
§ 1 Position and Posture by Acupuncture ················ 86
[1] Position of the Patient ························· 86
[2] Position of the Leg ························· 86
[3] Position of the Arm ························· 87
[4] Position of Practitioner ························· 88
§ 2 Management of Filiform Needle ················ 89
[1] Preliminary Massage ························· 89
[2] Disinfection ························· 89
[3] Skin Cutting and Needle Insertion ················ 89
A. Needle Tube Method ························· 89
B. Insertion without Needle Tube ················ 91
[4] Penetrating Needle into the Skin ················ 92
A. Direction of the Needle ························· 92
B. Prevention of Contamination ················ 93
C. Depth of Insertion ························· 93
D. Training of Skin Cutting and Needle Insertion ············ 93
§ 3 Getting KI (QI) ("Tokki" or "Hibiki") ················ 94
§ 4 Management of Intradermal Needle ················ 94
§ 5 Thumbtack Needle (En-pi-shin) ················ 95
Chapter 2 Stimulation and Supplementation-&-Draining ············ (97)
§ 1 Management of Needle for Supplementation and Draining ············ 97
[1] Type of Needle and Supplementation and Draining ············ 97

[2] Procedure of Insertion & Removing and Supplementation and Draining ···· 97
　　　[3] Stimulation and Supplementation & Draining ·· 98
　　§ 2 Method of Stimulation and Supplementation & Draining ························ 98
　　　[1] Retaining Needle Method ·· 98
　　　　A. Retaining Needle ·· 98
　　　　B. Intradermal Needle ·· 99
　　　　C. Thumbtack Needle (Drawing PinShaped Needle)s ······················ 99
　　　[2] Moxa Needle ·· 99
　　　[3] Manipulation ·· 99
　　　　Burning Mountain Method ·· 100
　　　　Penetrating Heaven Cooling Metod ·· 101
　　　[4] Bloodletting ·· 102
　　　　Bloodletting at WELL POINT ·· 102
　　　[5] Electro-acupuncture ·· 102
　　　[6] Acupoint Injection ·· 103
　　§ 3 Frequency of Acupuncture Therapy and Attention after Treatment ·········· 103
　　　[1] Frequency of Acupuncture Therapy ·· 103
　　　[2] Attention after Acupuncture Treatment ·· 104

PART 4　MY METHOD OF ACUPUNCTURE ·· (105)

　Chapter 1 Medical Examination for Acupuncture ·· (106)
　　§ 1 Inspection ·· 106
　　§ 2 Auscultation & Olfaction ·· 106
　　§ 3 Questioning ·· 106
　　§ 4 Palpation ·· 107
　　§ 5 Meridian Selection ·· 107
　　§ 6 Point Selection and Point Taking ·· 108
　Chapter 2 Treatment with Filiform Needle (Body Acupuncture) ···················· (109)
　　§ 1 Needle Insertion ·· 109
　　§ 2 Electro-acupuncture (Electric Acupuncture) ·· 109
　　　[1] Principled ·· 109
　　　　A. Supplementation & Draining with Electro-acupuncture ······················ 109
　　　　B. Balance of Stimulation ·· 110
　　　[2] Instruments for Electric Stimulation ·· 111
　　　　A. Structure and Merits of "Tokki" ·· 111
　　　　B. How to Operate "Tokki" ·· 112
　　　　C. Troubles of the Stimulator "Tokki" ·· 114
　　§ 3 Other Treatment with Filiform Needle (Body Acupuncture) ·························· 115
　　　[1] Retaining Needle and Manipulation ·· 115
　　　[2] Moxa Needle ·· 115
　Chapter 3 Other Acupuncture Therapies ·· (119)
　　§ 1 Intradermal Needle & Thumbtack Needle ·· 119

§ 2 Auricular Acupuncture ... 119
§ 3 Eyelid Acupuncture ... 120
§ 4 SSP ... 121
§ 5 Acupoint Injection ... 121
§ 6 Finger Pressure to Acupuncture Points ... 123
§ 7 Pasting Silver Grain or Magnetic Grain ... 123
Chapter 4 Appearance and Course of Effects ... 124

PART 5   COMPLICATIONS, SIDE EFFECTS & CASES OUT OF ACUPUNCTURE ... (126)

Chapter 1 Complications and Side Effects of Acupuncture ... (126)
§ 1 Leaving Needle ... 126
§ 2 Bleeding ... 126
§ 3 Needle Breakage ... 127
§ 4 Infection ... 127
[1] Contamination due to Imperfect Disinfection of the Skin ... 128
A. Dirty Skin ... 128
B. Unsuitable Disinfectants ... 128
C. Contaminated Disinfectants ... 128
[2] Contamination by Contaminated Needle Body ... 129
A. Contamination by Imperfect Disinfection of Needle ... 129
B. Contamination due to Improper Use of Needle ... 129
§ 5 Side Effects of Acupuncture ... 130
Chapter 2 Diseases out of Indication & Contraindications of Acupuncture ... (131)
§ 1 Diseases out of Indication of Acupuncture ... 131
§ 2 Cases out of Indication of Electro-acupuncture ... 132
§ 3 Contraindication of Intradermal acupuncture & Thumbtack Needle ... 132
§ 4 Contraindication of Acupuncture ... 133

PART 6   PRACTICE OF ACUPUNCTURE ... (134)

Chapter 1 Pain (Including Stiffness & Numbness) ... (134)
§ 1 General Rule ... 134
§ 2 Head (Except Face) ... 135
[1] Around the Center Line ... 136
[2] Outer Side of the Centre Line to Parietal Region ... 136
[3] Temporal- & Retro-auricular Region, Temple & Lateral Neck ... 137
[4] Forehead and Lateral Part of the Forehead ... 137
[5] Pain at Broad Area or Obscure Region ... 137
§ 3 Face and Mouth ... 138
[1] Eye ... 139
[2] Toothache ... 140
[3] Oral Cavity and/or Tongue ... 141
[4] Throat ... 141
[5] Face ... 142

  1) Lower Jaw 142
  2) Upper Jaw & Zygomatic Region 143
  3) Around the Nose 144
  4) Forehead 145
 § 4 Neck 146
  [1] Back of the Neck 146
  [2] Anterior &/or Lateral Part of the Neck 147
 § 5 Shoulder & Shoulder Joint 148
  [1] "Shoulder" 148
  [2] Around the Shoulder Joint 149
 § 6 Arm & Hand 151
  [1] General Rule 151
  [2] Elbow Joint 152
  [3] Hand Joint & Fingers 152
 § 7 Anterior- & Lateral Chest 152
 § 8 Abdominal Pain 154
  [1] Epigastrium (So Called "Stomachache") 155
  [2] Hypochondrium 155
  [3] Pain around Navel 155
  [4] Lower Abdomen 155
  [5] Inguinal Region 155
 § 9 Back & Lumbar Pain 156
 § 10 Sacral Region and around Gluteal Region 158
 § 11 Genital Area and around Anus 158
 § 12 Lower Extremity 160
  [1] Pain of the Leg 160
   1) Dorsal Side of the Leg 161
   2) Inner Side of the Leg 161
   3) Lateral Side of the Leg 161
   4) When the Localization of Pain is Too Wide or Indistinct 161
  [2] Pain in the Hip Joint 161
  [3] Pain in the Knee Joint 162
  [4] Pain of the Foot 163
 § 13 Pain of Malignant Tumor 163
Chapter 2 Acupuncture in Surgery, Orthopedics & Anesthesiology .... (165)
 § 1 Acupuncture Related to Operation 165
  [1] Acupuncture as Premedication 165
  [2] Acupuncture for Postoperative Pain 165
  [3] Acupuncture for Postoperative Paresis of Intestine 165
  [4] Aupuncture Anesthesia 166
 § 2 Acupuncture Therapy for Fresh Injury 167

    [1] General Fresh Injury (Wound, Fracture etc.) ……………… 167
    [2] Compression Fracture of Vertebra ……………………………… 167
  § 3 Refractory Fistula ……………………………………………………… 168
  § 4 Whiplash Syndrome …………………………………………………… 168
    [1] Method of Treatment ………………………………………………… 168
    [2] Effect and Process of Acupuncture Therapy …………………… 170
    [3] Acupoint Injection for Whiplash Syndrome ……………………… 171
  § 5 Cervicobrachial Syndrome & Thoracic Outlet Syndrome ……… 171
  § 6 Lumber & Back Pain …………………………………………………… 171
  § 7 Spinal Canal Stenosis ………………………………………………… 172
  § 8 Acupuncture Therapy for Articular Pain …………………………… 172
Chapter 3 Diseases of Nervous System …………………………………… (174)
  § 1 Central Nervous System ……………………………………………… 174
  § 2 Neuralgia ………………………………………………………………… 174
    [1] Trigeminal Neuralgia and Diseases with Similar Symptom …… 174
    [2] Intercostal Neuralgia ………………………………………………… 176
    [3] Sciatica ………………………………………………………………… 176
    [4] Post-herpetic Neuralgia (PHN) ……………………………………… 176
    [5] Diabetic Neuralgia …………………………………………………… 179
  § 3 Motor Paralysis ………………………………………………………… 179
    [1] Facial Nerve Paralysis ……………………………………………… 179
    [2] Recurrent Nerve Paralysis ………………………………………… 181
    [3] Motor Paralysis of Extremities (According to Mr. AOYAGI's oral teaching) ‥ 182
    [4] Myasthenia Gravis …………………………………………………… 183
Chapter 4 Acupuncture in Psychiatric Area ……………………………… (184)
  § 1 Depressive State ……………………………………………………… 184
  § 2 Somatoform Disorder ………………………………………………… 184
Chapter 5 Diseases of Digestive Organ & Metabolic Diseases …………… (185)
  § 1 Nausea and Vomiting ………………………………………………… 185
  § 2 Hiccup …………………………………………………………………… 185
  § 3 Dehydrated Feeling of the Mouth …………………………………… 186
  § 4 Constipation …………………………………………………………… 186
  § 5 Obesity ………………………………………………………………… 187
    [1] Method of Treatment ………………………………………………… 187
    [2] Meal during Treatment ……………………………………………… 188
    [3] Process of the Effect ………………………………………………… 188
    [4] Attention by This Treatment ………………………………………… 188
Chapter 6 Diseases of Respiratory Organs ……………………………… (190)
  § 1 Bronchial Asthma ……………………………………………………… 190
  § 2 Diseases with Asthma-like Symptom ……………………………… 191
Chapter 7 Acupuncture in Gynecology …………………………………… (192)

§ 1 Dysmenorrhea 192
§ 2 Menopausal Disorder 193
§ 3 Emesis (Morning Sickness) 193
§ 4 Painless Delivery 194

Chapter 8 Acupuncture in Dermatology .... (195)
§ 1 General Rule for Acupuncture for Dermal Disease 195
§ 2 Urticaria 196
§ 3 Erosion around Artificial Anus 196
§ 4 Fresh Herpes Zoster 197
  [1] Method of treatment 197
  [2] Meridian & Point Selection 197
  [3] Effect of Acupuncture and the Course 198
  [4] Frequency and Length of Treatment 199
§ 5 Atopic Dermatitis 199
§ 6 Palmoplantar Pustulosis 199

Chapter 9 Acupuncture for Complaints of Ear, Nose and Throat .... (200)
§ 1 Acupuncture for Disorder of the Ear 200
  [1] Meridians and Points Related to Ear 200
  [2] Pain of the Ear 201
  [3] Tinnitus, Dizziness, Hearing Loss 201
    A. Hearing Loss 201
    B. Tinnitus 202
    C. Dizziness 203
  [4] Symptoms of the Nose 203
  [5] Pollinosis 204
  [6] Complaints of Pharyngo-Laryngeal Region 204

Chapter 10 Acupuncture in Ophthalmology .... (206)
§ 1 General Rule 206
§ 2 Pain of the Eye 207
§ 3 Diplopia 207
§ 4 Ocular Hypertension 207

Chapter 11 Acupuncture for Urinary Organ and Impotence .... (208)
§ 1 Dysuria 208
§ 2 Urolithiasis 208
§ 3 Impotence 208
§ 4 IgA Nephropathy 208

Chapter 12 Allergic or Autoimmune Disorders .... (209)
§ 1 General Rule 209
§ 2 Bronchial Asthma 210
§ 3 Pollinosis (Allergic Rhinitis and Conjunctivitis) 210
§ 4 Chronic Urticaria 212

§ 5 Atopic Dermatitis ·· 213
§ 6 Palmoplantar Pustulosis ·· 213
§ 7 IgA Nephropathy ··· 214
§ 8 Myasthenia Gravis ·· 216
§ 9 Sjögren's Syndrome ·· 217
§ 10 Fibromyalgia ··· 218
§ 11 Alopecia Areata ··· 218
INDEX ·· 220

PART 1

INTRODUCTION
— OUTLINE OF ACUPUNCTURE —

Chapter 1   Principle and Characteristics of Acupuncture
§ 1   Principle of Acupuncture

Acupuncture is a therapeutic method by which needles are inserted into certain points of the skin to give suitable stimulation through the needles. Some of its mechanism of effect is clearly explained by the Occidental methods as "Gate Control Theory" or "Endorphin Theory" etc. But various effects of acupuncture are not elucidated by these theories yet.

On the other hand, there are classic principles of acupuncture. From the viewpoint of Occidental Medicine, they may appear absurd because of lack of any evidence. But by the acupuncture therapy, on the assumption that these principles are true, extremely excellent effects, often better than Occidental Medicine, are obtained. I would like to admit the classic theories free from bias.

The principles are as described below:

1. There are "Meridians" in the body, and "KI$^{(Jp.)}$ (QI$^{(Ch)}$) and "BLOOD" flow through Meridians.
   KI(QI) is something having its function but no shape. "BLOOD" flows through body (meridians) like blood, but it is not same as "Occidental concept of blood").
2. When the flow of KI(QI) & BLOOD become unfavorable, the body becomes ill.
3. By insertion of needle to certain points to give some stimulation, the flow of KI(QI) & BLOOD can be affected.
4. Ill body can be cured by stimulating some points with needle, which normalizes the flow of KI(QI) & BLOOD.
5. There are two types of disorder in the flow of KI(QI) & BLOOD, namely Deficiency (lack of correct KI(QI)) and Excess (meridians are full of pathogen KI(QI)).
6. Methods of therapy is as follows:
   Supplementation for Deficiency: To sapply correct KI(QI)
   Draining for Excess: To remove pathogen KI(QI)

Those who are educated by Occidental Medicine may feel puzzled with the terms and theories of acupuncture. But, at this stage, please accept the concept of predecessors humbly.

§ 2   Merits and Demerits of Acupuncture

[1] Merits of Acupuncture

The following merits of acupuncture are known.

1) Acupuncture is Simple and Easy to Perform, Less Invasive, and Quite Effective.

Acupuncture therapy can be practiced with a few needles and small dose of disinfectant. Large instrument for sterilization of the utensils is not necessary, and by using disposable needles, the instrument for sterilization of the waste is not necessary. Large space is not needed for treatment of one patient because necessary instruments are not large. The only necessary special equipment is ventilator for moxibustion. For electro-acupuncture, a special instrument is necessary. But it is not so big, and not so expensive. Everything needed to acupuncture is smaller in size and in expenditure. This is a marked merit of acupuncture therapy.

The pain due to needling puncture is unavoidable. Acupuncture needles, however, are so fine, that the pain is much less than that due to usual injection. Except willful children or those who have excessive reflex like patients with cerebral disorders, there is no problems to practice acupuncture therapy.

2) Effects Appear Promptly

Usually the effects come to light after one or two treatment, excepting for a few cases such as motor paralysis or post-herpetic neuralgia and the like. The quick showing of the effect will encourage patient to continue treatment.

3) Effective Therapy is Possible without Definite Diagnosis

In Occidental Medicine, radical treatment without definite diagnosis is impossible. And there are some diseases that have no treatment method available even though the name of disease is identified. In Oriental Medicine, the treatment is performed according to the patient's "Shou[(Jp.)]" (symptom complex in the meaning of Oriental Medicine). Thus, treatment can be performed as if the name of the disease is not identified. Or rather, strategy of treatment is different from the diagnosis of the disease in the meaning of Occidental Medicine.

This fact does not mean "Treatment of Oriental medicine is only symptomatic therapy". For example, for many kinds of cold or influenza, Kampo[(Jp.)] treatment under correct Oriental diagnosis produces more delicate and better effect than Occidental Medicine.

In Occidental Medicine, treatment of pain must be performed under strictly correct diagnosis. Treatment of pain without diagnosis of disease is only a symptomatic therapy. Thereby diagnosis as well as treatment is often very difficult. On the other hand, acupuncture therapy is performed according to the "Shou[(Jp.)]" of the patient. For the patient with same "Shou", same treatment is given independent of the Occidental diagnosis. If the patient's "Shou" is different, different treatment is given each, even if the Occidental diagnosis is same. Effects are often superior to Occidental Medicine.

Of course, diagnosis of "Shou$^{(Jp.)}$" is always necessary, and it demands some training. But it is much easier and less expensive than Occidental training

This merit contains a kind of risk. What needs to be paid attention is that acupuncture is very effective. Especially, acupuncture for pain sedation, most of pain is sedated (often it vanishes). Then, the patient sometimes misunderstands that the disease has cured.

Because of the excellent effect of acupuncture, there is another problem that patient's important symptoms can be buried, and it can mislead diagnosis. By acupuncture therapy, we must never be content with the effect of acupuncture, but we must make effort for definite diagnosis in the meaning of Occidental Medicine.

4) Broad Range of Indications

Pain or stiffness is good target for acupuncture. But there are plenty of other diseases and symptoms which can be cured more easily by acupuncture therapy, sometimes more efficiently than Occidental Medicine.

5) Less Side Effects and Complications

Kampo medicine (Japanese herbal medicine) has less side effects than Occidental medicine. Acupuncture has much less side effects than Kampo medicine. Unavoidable pain by needling and fatigue due to too strong stimulation or bathing after acupuncture or overwork on the next day of the treatment may trigger rather unique minor side effect.

The complication that most frequently appears is subcutaneous bleeding. Complete prevention of this "complication" is almost impossible. But it is rather unusual, and it surely disappears at most in a few weeks. In my method, treatment region is mainly peripheral parts of extremities. So, this complication seldom causes cosmetic problem.

Other possible complications such as infection, pneumothorax, needle breakage or burn by moxa needle etc. are almost completely evadable by normal attention.

[2] Demerits of Acupuncture

There are, however, some demerits of acupuncture as described below.

1) Training is necessary

Training is indispensable in all the fields of medical practice. But acupuncture is a field out of the Occidental Medicine. So, for ordinary medical doctors or dentists this training may be a big barrier.

2) Effects vary markedly according to the ability of the practitioner

It is quite reasonable to say that the effect of therapy by an unskilled practitioner is not good. But the fact that "Unskilled practitioner hardly gives good effects" seems much more evident by acupuncture than the result of surgical operation even for early stage gastric cancer by unskilled surgeon.

3) Risk of delaying or misleading diagnosis

Effects of acupuncture are often quite excellent at removing pains or other complaints of patients, so that the patient miscomprehend to the degree that the causative disease is completely cured by acupuncture. And the patient sometimes discontinues necessary therapy. "Excellent effects" can hide important symptoms, and correct diagnosis can be delayed or misled by excellent effect of acupuncture.

4) Adverse reaction to needle puncture

Pain of needle insertion is inevitable though it is usually much lighter than the usual injection pain. There are some methods of painless acupuncture. But some patients feel "needle puncture" just like surgical operation. In such a case, just give the patient finger pressure to the relevant acupuncture point, which is fairly painful. Then tell the patient that acupuncture is less painful than the finger pressure, which often persuade patients successfully

5) Low economic efficiency

Usually practicing acupuncture therapy takes time. To treat many patients, a spacious room is necessary. When doctors or dentists practice acupuncture by themselves, these factors may be the greatest barrier.

Chapter 2   Indications and Methods of Acupuncture

§ 1   Indications of Acupuncture

Acupuncture is very effective in the treatment of many diseases and symptoms.
Even just limited to my own experiences there are many indications as mentioned below:
1) Pain, stiffness, itching, numbness.
2) Diseases in which pain plays a serious role.
   (Whiplash syndrome, Herpes Zoster, Dysmenorrhea etc.)
3) So called unidentified complaints
4) Bronchial asthma
5) Gynecological diseases (Dysmenorrhea, Emesis, Menopausal Disorders etc.)
6) Complaints of the nose
   (Nasal obstruction, Rhinorrhea, Olfactory disorder, Pollinosis etc.)
7) Tinnitus, Vertigo, Hearing loss etc.
8) Complaints of the eye
   (Pain, Diplopia, Visual disorder, Ocular hypertension, Pollinosis etc.)
9) Dermal diseases
   (Herpes Zoster, Urticaria, Atopic dermatitis, Palmoplantar Pustulosis etc.)
10) Hiccup
11) IgA Nephropathy
12) Neural paralysis
13) Obesity
14) Inflammation, Refractory fistula

In addition, I have some effective case of diabetes mellitus or myasthenia gravis etc., and in many textbooks of acupuncture, vast number of indications of acupuncture are enumerated.

§ 2   Methods of Acupuncture

Basically, acupuncture is to insert needles to suitable points to give suitable stimulation through the needle.

To determine the points to be treated is called "Point Selection". In classic literatures, 361 (or 365) points are given on head, neck, trunk (chest, abdomen and back) and extremities. Acupuncture using these points is called "body acupuncture". Recently, additional points at the ear, head and hand are proposed which are called "auricular acupuncture", "scalp acupuncture" and "hand acupuncture" respectively. In my practice, body acupuncture is most commonly practiced. Sometimes auricular acupuncture is also used with body acupuncture.

[1] Principles of Acupuncture Therapy

Acupuncture is performed on the two principles.
1. To select the local points of complaints, and treat them mainly to remove the existing complaints.
2. To treat the patient adjusting the patient's imbalance of the whole body or the flow of meridians.

The former is called "symptomatic treatment", and the latter "root treatment". For the root treatment, the most important thing is to adjust imbalances among the meridians. Thus, it is sometimes called "Meridian Treatment". But "Meridian Treatment" has other definition. So called "Meridian Treatment" is one method of "Root Treatment" in the broad sense.

In the most of schools, treatment of "Root Treatment" or "Meridian Treatment" starts from "diagnosis in the meaning of Oriental Medicine" of the patient. This diagnosis is to judge the present state of the patient by elaborating through inspection, auscultation & olfaction, questioning and palpation etc., and adding pattern identification of KI[JP.](QI[Ch.])/BLOOD/WATER, and careful consideration of generating-&-destructive relationship of "FIVE ELEMENTS" etc. Thus the diagnosis of ORGANS to be treated is given. After elucidating the relevant ORGANs, meridians to be treated are decided.

According to this method, the meridian to be treated is decided after determining the "SHOU[JP.] (SYMPTOMs)" of ORGANS. This is very complicated and extremely difficult. It may be almost impossible to practice this method properly by self-education, without good master.

[2] Methods of Stimulation

To insert needle itself is a kind of stimulation. There are many kinds of stimulation after insertion of needles, as mentioned below.

1) Single Needle Technique

This is a method to insert needles to adequate depth without twisting, and then to remove the needle immediately. By changing the direction of insertion or the speed of insertion & removal, this method can be used both for supplementation and draining.

2) Free-hand Regular Method

This is a method to twist the needle. Needle is given twisting by insertion &/or at the end of insertion &/or by removing. This method can be used both for supplementation and draining according to the style of torsion.

3) Sparrow Pecking Method

This is a method to give a repeated stimulation of inserting and lifting to a very limited range through the needle, after insertion to a suitable depth. The pattern of this stimulation resembles the movement of a sparrow pecking food.

4) Retaining Needle

This is a method to leave the inserted needle for some time. This method is used mainly for supplementation but draining is not impossible. Intradermal acupuncture including drawing pin type intradermal needle (= thumbtack needle), which is very shallow acupuncture (unique in Japan) may be a kind of this retaining needle method.

5) Intermittent Insertion Method

This is a method to move the needle forward intermittently after the insertion.

6) Vibration

This is a method to give vibration to needle by flipping or rubbing the needle.

7) Scattering Acupuncture

This is a method to insert many needles superficially to the part or around the complaint. The method to insert single needle repeatedly and in different directions is also called by this name.

8) Depletion (Blood Letting)

This is a method to cause bleeding by using a thick needle. Sometimes cupping is used for this purpose. This method is used for draining.

9) Manipulation

This is a method combining the above mentioned techniques 2), 3), 5). This method can be used both for supplementation and draining.

10) Moxa Needle

This is a method to burn moxa attached on the handle of the needle. This method is used mainly for supplementation.

11) Electro-acupuncture

This is a method to give electric stimulation through retained needles. This method can be used both for supplementation and draining. This method has excellent merits such as less pain and less troubles than above mentioned manipulation method, possibility of long time treatment and quantitative comparison etc.

[3] Acupuncture without Acupuncture Needle

Some techniques may be regarded as a kind of acupuncture although acupuncture needle is not inserted, because these methods can treat the relevant diseases or symptoms under the same principle as that of acupuncture.

1) Contact Needling (Dermal Acupuncture or Pediatric Acupuncture)

This method uses acupuncture needle just to touch with the tip of the needle without insertion. This is used mainly for children, but it can be used for extremely sensitive adults. For this method, some specific instruments are provided.

2) SSP[5]

This method uses a metallic conical object to give an electric stimulation to the patient. Stimulation is given by applying the sharp-pointed tip of the instrument on the acupuncture point.

3) TENS (transcutaneous electrical nerve stimulation) is similar to SSP, used in the same way as SSP. Its tip, however, is not sharp pointed.

4) Acupoint Injection

This method is to inject some substance to acupuncture points (acupoints). The idea is to replace acupuncture needle with injection needle and to use injection as stimulation. Any substance that can be used subcutaneously or intramuscularly (such as physiological saline solution, vitamins, anodynes or opiates etc.) can be used. Excellent effects are obtained with any substance. In my practice, it is performed under completely same idea as that of electro-aupuncture. This method should be considered as a kind of acupuncture.

5) Finger Pressure Therapy

This is a method to give patients finger pressure at the patient's acupuncture point. It is fairly painful, but sometimes very effective.

6) Stimulation of Static Electricity

This method is to stimulate acupuncture points with high voltage static electricity. For this method some instruments are commercially available.

7) Silver- or Magnet- Grain

This is a method to put silver-grated grain or magnet grain on the acupuncture points. The effect is not so evident.

8) Laser Acupuncture

This is a method to apply laser beam to acupuncture points.

Among methods mentioned above, electro-acupuncture ([2]-11) is the basic method of my acupuncture. Additionally, retaining needle ([2]-4) including drawing-pin shaped needle (thumbtack needle), manipulation ([2]-9), moxa needle ([2]-10) and acupoint injection ([3]-4) are mostly used in my practice. Sometimes finger pressure therapy is also used as the test.

Chapter 3 Acupuncture Needles

Since ancient days, various kinds of needles have been used. In Reisuu[Jp.] (霊枢)[1], nine kinds of needles are described with their indications. Today, many kinds of "needles", including the instruments of pediatric acupuncture or static electricity stimulation etc., are in use. In my practice, (except injection needle for acupoint injection) only three kinds of needles, namely filiform needle, intradermal needle and thumbtack needle (drawing pin type needle) are commonly used. A range of diseases and symptoms can be treated with them only.

According to previously described principle, only these three types of needles are explained in this book.

§ 1 Filiform Needle (毫鍼 Goushin[Jp.])

Filiform needle is the most typical and most frequently used acupuncture needle. It consists of a handle and straight metallic wire whose one end is sharpened and the other end is buried in the handle. The wire part (called "needle body") is made of metal (gold, silver or stainless steel, or gold-or-silver plated stainless steel), and the handle part is made of plastic or metal (usually stainless steel). They are jointed together with glue or by soldering or welding or pressure bonding. In my practice, the needle is exclusively made of stainless steel attached with welded or pressure bonded metallic handle, because of the convenience for electric stimulation and moxa needle. Chinese needles are generally thicker and longer than the Japanese ones, and the shape of handle is different and longer than Japanese needles. The handle of Chinese needle has a projection at the end of the handle which does not allow the use of needle tube. It is quite unwelcome, especially for beginners.

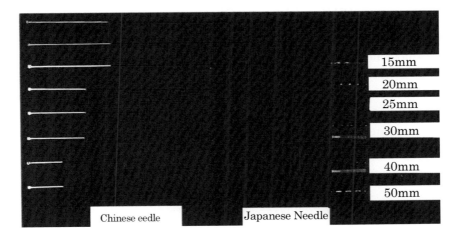

Fig.2 Filiform Needle

Size of Filiform Needle

1. Diameter

Japanese needles are much finer than the Chinese ones.

Size of Japanese needles commonly used are of eleven types with the diameter, range from 0.14mm (No.0 or size 14) to 0.34 mm (No.10 or size 34) in diameter. The difference of one number is 0.02mm in diameter, and the size of needle is named by hundred times of its diameter in millimeter. In my method, mainly two size of needles are used, namely No.3 (Size 18) needle for supplementation, and No.5 (size 24) needle for draining.

2. Length

Length of the needle is named according to the length of the needle body. In Japan, formerly it was called by Japanese measures (Sun, 1Sun ≒ 3.03cm). Recently "meter system" is widely used, and now the size of needle is called by both naming. Today, in Japan, needles ranging from 1.5cm (0.5sun = 5Bu) to 10cm (3Sun) are available. In my method, needle of 4cm (1.3Sun) and 5cm (1.6Sun) in length are mainly used. For auricular acupuncture, 1.5cm, 2.0cm or 2.5cm in length is used. Needle of 2.0cm in length is most convenient for auricular acupuncture and eyelid acupuncture.

For acupuncture anesthesia, thicker (over 0.34mm in diameter) and very long needle is required. For that purpose, Chinese needles may be more convenient.

Thickness of the needle has some relation with supplementation & draining, i.e. finer needles are used for supplementation and thicker needle for draining.

The difference of 0.04mm in diameter is visually difficult to identify. In order to distinguish the two, it is much easier to distinguish them by the length. So, in my practice, finer and longer needle (No.3, 5cm) is used for supplementation, and thicker and shorter needle (No.5, 4cm) for draining.

§ 2 Intradermal Needle (in Narrow Sense)[7]

Intradermal acupuncture is a method to insert very short needle into the epidermis almost horizontally, and to retain it for several days. Insertion must be very shallow, at most before reaching the layer of subcutaneous tissue. Needle of this type is fine (No.1 or No.2) and short (3mm to 10mm) and it has a very short handle. The merit of this needle is possibility of both supplementation and draining by treatment. But the insertion and retaining technique is not so easy. So, recently this needle is seldom used.

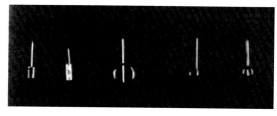

Fig.3 Intradermal Needle

§ 3　Thumbtack Type Needle (En-pishin$^{(Jp.)}$) (Thumbtack Needle) (Fig.4)

The shape of this needle of the original type is like that of drawing pin. Length of the needle is from 3mm to 10mm or so. En-pi-shin$^{(Jp.)}$ means round skin-needle.

Recently, needles of a new type with same function is commercially available. The needle is pasted on a small round sticking plaster, sterilized and packed separately. Needle of this type is very convenient to use, and it is painless. It can be used in nearly the same as the previous intradermal needles. Today, in my practice, needles of this design are mostly used instead of intradermal needle.

Very short needles can be retained within the epidermal layer almost without the risk of infection even if it is left for several days. So, long needle over 0.6mm in length are not recommended

It has some demerits. That is:
1. It is doubtful if it can be used for draining (but it is often very effective).
2. Accurate insertion is very difficult.

It seems apparently very easy. But exact hitting is essentially requested, and it is impossible to touch the point after disinfection. "Getting KI$^{(Jp.)}$(QI$^{(Ch.)}$)" seldom appears by insertion. The practitioner must visually locate the point. This may be the most difficult method of acupuncture (without point detector).

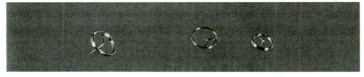

Original Type

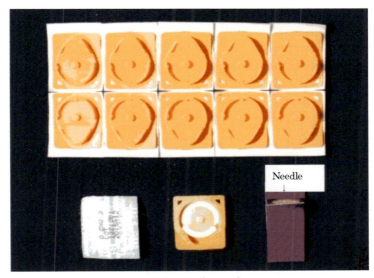

New Type (0.3mm)

Fig.4　Thumbtack Needle

Chapter 4   Meridian and Acupuncture Point

§ 1   Meridian & Acupuncture Point (Acupoint or Point)

On the human body surface, there are many particular points connected with ORGANs. These points are called "Tsubo(Jp.)" or Acupuncture Point or Point or Acupoint. There are points, resembling each other to form a group. Connecting those points of similar character, some line, like a meridian, is observed on the surface of the body. By needle insertion or stimulation, occasionally some unusual sensation appears. When some medicine is injected at a point, sometimes the patient feels as if something flows along the meridian. This kind of sensation is called "Meridian Phenomenon". The concept of "Meridian" may originate in such experiences.

According to the classic literatures, there are some groups of meridians in the body, through which KI(Jp.)(QI(Ch.)) and Ketsu(Jp.) (BLOOD) flow. When their flow is smooth, the body is healthy, whereas when it becomes irregular, the body gets ill.

Someone said that there was a person who could see meridians on the surface of the body. However, nobody could prove the presence of meridians on solid scientific evidences.

Any acupuncture practitioners scarcely neglect the acupuncture points. Yet there are acupuncturists who doubt the existence of meridians, and they practice acupuncture ignoring meridians.

Among those who believe the existence of meridians, their opinions are various. Someone says that the meridian may be the blood vessel, others say that it may be the lymph duct. The manner of spreading of meridian phenomenon or its spreading speed suggest me that the meridian is a kind of pathway of very fine non-myelinated nerve fiber. Anyway, none of those stories have sufficient scientific evidence. It is, however, undoubted fact that acupuncture therapy under the classic meridian theory produces excellent effects, sometimes much better than Occidental Medicine. It may be the best way to accept the classic theory as it is.

Many textbooks on acupuncture say that "The meridian connects with some ORGAN". "Connect with something" may be analogous to the meaning of the term of "control of the nerve" by anatomy in Occidental Medicine. That is, "to distribute to some organ and to influence on the function of the organ". ORGAN is not the same as the anatomical organ. They can be completely different. In Chinese books, pathways of meridians are represented like "general chart" and distribute to the anatomical organs of the same name of ORGANs. It sounds unreasonable to me, though the idea that "meridians exists not only on the surface of the body but also in the deep part of the body" can be agreed. Indeed, the real meridians may exist in the deep part of the body, and the meridians of body surface may be just their projection.

Even very shallow acupuncture is almost always effective. Injection to acupuncture point creates a sensation of flow along the correspondent meridian. From these facts, functional activity of points of body surface is evident. But "getting KI(Jp.)(QI(Ch.))"(explained later) is felt better rather by deeper insertion. This fact may suggest that the real meridians are situated not on the body surface but deep in the body, and the points of the body surface may be the connecting points with the corresponding meridians.

The relation between the ORGAN and the acupuncture point is: according to the late Dr. MANAKA, similar to the relation between a country and its embassy or consulate. It is a quite excellent metaphor.

Meridians (and collaterals) are composed of 12 pairs of main meridians and 8 extra meridians. (There are other analogous pathways called "muscle meridian" or "divergent meridian". But as I have no chance to use them, these meridians are not described in this book.)

Main meridians are where "K$^{(Jp.)}$I(QI$^{(Ch.)}$) and Ketsu$^{(Jp.)}$(BLOOD) flow through like water flows though the river, whereas extra meridians play a role of flood retarding basin or marsh or lake to support the smooth flow of the river. Among the extra meridians, GOVERNOR VESSEL (GV) and CONCEPTION VESSEL (CV) have their own acupuncture points, and they are regarded to be specifically important. Accordingly, 12 pairs of main meridians, together with these two important extra meridians, are called "Fourteen Meridians".

In my practice, extra meridians are not so frequently used except GOVERNOR VESSEL (GV) and CONCEPTION VESSEL (CV), although many acupuncturists use those extra meridians as important acupuncture points. It may be better to use those extra meridians as well. But it is also true that without the use of those extra meridians, excellent effects are obtained in wide range.

Each meridian has its own name. Meridians are called by the name of IN$^{(Jp.)}$(YIN$^{(Ch.)}$) or YO-U$^{(Jp.)}$ (YANG$^{(Ch.)}$) ORGAN which corresponds to the meridian. Each meridian has its character of IN (YIN) or YO-U (YANG). Meridian which has name of IN (YIN) ORGAN is IN(YIN) meridian, and meridian which has name of YO-U (YANG) ORGAN is YO-U (YANG) meridian. YO-U(YANG) meridians (except STOMACH Meridian) pass through the area on which the sun shines, namely the back side of the trunk, the extensor side of upper extremities and back-and-out side of the lower extremities, whereas IN(YIN)

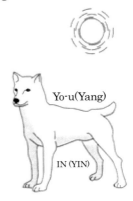

Fig.5 Concept of IN(YIN) and YO-U(YANG)

meridians pass through shadow part, namely the abdominal side of the trunk, the flexor side of the upper extremities and the inner side of the lower extremities (Fig.5).

The character "IN(YIN)" and "YO-U(YANG)" of meridians is very important by acupuncture treatment (it will be mentioned later).

ORGAN and organ is, as if the name is the same, hardly considered to be equal because their function is often extremely different like SPLEEN and spleen.

However, the name of the meridians is convenient to estimate the character IN$^{(Jp.)}$ or YO-U$^{(Jp.)}$ of the meridian. Meridians (also ORGANs) which have the name of parenchymatous organs (except PERICARDIUM and HEART) are IN(YIN) meridians or ORGANs, and that of hollow organs are YO-U(YANG) meridians or ORGANs.

§ 2 Flow of KI$^{(Jp.)}$ (QI$^{(Ch.)}$) and Ketsu$^{(Jp.)}$ (BLOOD) in the Meridian

The meridian is considered to start as LUNG Meridian which rises from "Chuushou$^{(Jp.)}$" (MIDDLE ENERGIZER), located near CV$_{12}$, which is situated at the middle of xiphoid process and the navel. LUNG Meridian starts from Chuushou$^{(Jp.)}$ and, via LARGE INTESTINE → entrance of STOMACH → diaphragm → LUNG → front of the shoulder joint → radial side of the upper extremity → the end of the thumb, and links with LARGE INTESTINE Meridian. LARGE INTESTINE Meridian links with STOMACH meridian, and then the meridian's flow with the following order: →SPLEEN Meridian, → HEART Meridian → SMALL INTESTINE Meridian → BLADDER Meridian → KIDNEY Meridian → PERICARDIUM Meridian → TRIPLE ENERGIZER Meridian → GALLBLADDER Meridian → LIVER Meridian. After that, it goes back to LUNG Meridian. KI$^{(Jp.)}$QI$^{(Ch.)}$ and BLOOD are considered to circulate in this order through meridian. Direction of this flow is very important for the acupuncture treatment. Putting it simply, the direction of flow of IN$^{(Jp.)}$(YIN$^{(Ch.)}$) meridians is upward and that of YO-U$^{(Jp.)}$ (YANG$^{(Ch.)}$) meridian downward. It is very simple. But beginners often misunderstand the flow in the upper extremity. "Up" or "down" is meant by holding-up style (Fig.6).

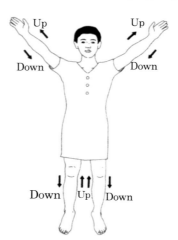

Fig.6   Direction of Flow "IN up, YO-U down"

The direction of extra meridians is not clear. The direction of GOVERNOR VESSEL and CONCEPTION VESSEL, the routes of which are vertical, is obscure even in classic literature. Under the hypothesis that "the function of extra meridians is like marsh or lake", it may be rather reasonable that the direction of flow in extra meridians is not defined.

§ 3 Fourteen Meridians and Acupuncture Therapy

In many classic books, including Reisuu$^{(Jp.)}$ (霊枢), detailed description of meridians are given (Hereafter,the meridians of this sort are reffered to "classic meridian"). Routes of classic meridians are different from those in general meridian charts (Fig.1). The difference between classic literatures and general charts are as shown below.
1) In the general charts, the routes in the deep part of the body are not shown.
2) The meridians in the classic literatures have branches. In the general charts, only STOMACH(ST) Meridian and BLADDER(BL) Meridian have branches and others do not. Moreover, in some meridians of the general charts, some parts (sometimes whole !) of the chief meridians are omitted.
3) Some routes of classic literature extend further beyond the end of the meridian of the general charts.
4) Routes of meridians of classic literature and those of the general charts are not always the same.

Some of classic meridians have highly complicated routes. The beginners, for example, may not comprehended the classic routes of GALLBLADDER Meridia at one glance.

Many cases can be treated according to the general chart with excellent effects. In many cases, however, better effects are obtained by the treatment following the classic literature. Therefore, in this book, routes of both of general chart and classic literature are given. The relation to acupuncture therapy are explained in detail.

[1] LUNG Meridian (LU)

> **Outline of the Meridian**
> LUNG Meridian (LU) starts at the upper abdominal area, and via LARGE INTESTINE → entrance of STOMACH → diaphragm → LUNG → front of the shoulder joint → radial side of the upper extremity. From here it arrives at the end of the thumb where it connects with LARGE INTESTINE Meridian.

Details of the Routes

LUNG Meridian starts at Chuushou$^{(Jp.)}$ (MIDDLE ENERGIZER), which is at the middle of the area between xiphoid process and navel. It goes down to LARGE INTESTINE (LI), turns back to the entrance of STOMACH, passes through the diaphragm and belongs to LUNG, then it comes out in front of the shoulder joint. From here, it goes along the radial side of the flexor side of upper extremity, and reaches the end of the thumb. One branch separates at LU$_7$, which goes to the end of the index finger, connecting with LARGE INTESTINE Meridian there.

In the general charts, only the route from LU$_1$ to the end of the thumb is shown.

16   PART 1 INTRODUCTION – OUTLINE OF ACUPUNCTURE –

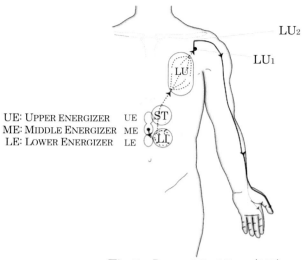

Fig. 7   LUNG Meridian (LU)

LUNG Meridian and Acupuncture Therapy
Points of LUNG Meridian are used for the following cases with good effects.
1) Treatment of the complaints of shoulder joint
   Many patients suffering from shoulder pain have complaints at the front of the shoulder joint where LUNG Meridian passes. Most cases need treatment of LUNG Meridian.
2) Treatment of complaints of the lung
   LUNG Meridian belongs to LUNG. The word "belong to" is used in the same meaning of "connect with". LUNG and anatomical lung are not exactly the same, though the function of LUNG is partially similar to that of lung. Treatment of the points of LUNG Meridian is usually effective for toss, asthma or dyspnea and the like.
3) Treatment of constipation or diarrhea
   LUNG Meridian belongs to LARGE INTESTINE. For the treatment of constipation or diarrhea, points of LARGE INTESTINE Meridian (LI) are usually used. But the treatment on the points of LUNG Meridian is sometimes effective.
4) Treatment of dermal diseases
   "Skin and hair belong to LUNG" is a unique concept of Oriental Medicine. Actually, treatment of LUNG Meridian is often surprisingly effective for the dermal diseases such as itching, urticaria, atopic dermatitis or palmoplantar pustulosis and the like.

[2] LARGE INTESTINE Meridian (LI)

Outline of the Meridian
LARGE INTESTINE Meridian starts from the tip of the index finger. It goes along the outer radial side of the upper extremity, and arrives at the shoulder. Then it divides into two routes. The chief one goes down through LUNG to LARGE INTESTINE, and a branch goes up via neck and around mouth to nose.

Details of the Routes
LARGE INTESTINE Meridian (LI) starts from the tip of the index finger. The route up to shoulder (Supraclavicular Fossa) is: origin (tip of the index finger) → radial side of index finger → between 1st and 2nd metacarpus → radial side of the arm → shoulder → GV_{14}, (between 7th cervical vertebra and 1st thoracic vertebra) → shoulder → ST_{12} (around middle of the clavicle). At ST_{12} the meridian divides into two routes. The chief meridian goes down, connects with LUNG, passes through diaphragm, and reaches LARGE INTESTINE. The other route (branch) goes from ST_{12} → front of the neck → through cheek → teeth of lower jaw → around mouth → and ends at the opposite side of the nose.

The route in general chart is the same as that in the classic literature up to the shoulder. Thereafter, however, the route of general chart is strikingly different from that of classic literature.

(According to SAWADA's chart, this meridian runs from LI_{20} to TE_{20}, whereas Reisuu(Jp.) (霊枢) says that "It ends at the side of nasal hole". The description of Reisuu is adopted here.)

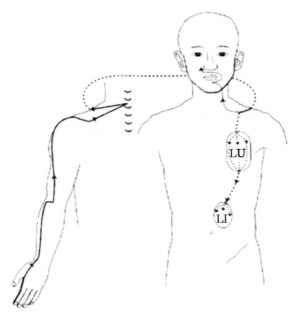

Fig.8 LARGE INTESTINE Meridian

The route of the general charts is different from that in the classic literature in the following points. General chart is:
1) The route to GV_{14} is not shown.
2) The route does not pass supraclavicular fossa.
3) Chief meridian that reaches LARGE INTESTINE via LUNG is absent.
4) Route from shoulder to nose is shown as the chief meridian.

LARGE INTESTINE Meridian and Acupuncture Therapy

Points of LARGE INTESTINE Meridian is used in the following cases with good effects.
1) Treatment of pain of the extensor side of the upper extremity.
2) Treatment of pain &/or movement disorder of shoulder joints
3) Treatment of pain at the anterior part of the neck
4) Treatment of complaints of the face and the teeth
5) Treatment of complaints related to the nose
   (Pain, Nasal Obstruction, Rhinorrhea, Pollinosis, Olfactory Disorder etc.)

The above mentioned cases are about the complaints of the spots where LARGE INTESTINE Meridian passes.

6) Treatment of abnormal intestinal peristalsis such as constipation, diarrhea, postoperative intestinal paralysis.

The LARGE INTESTINE Meridian belongs to LARGE INTESTINE. Some functions of LARGE INTESTINE resemble those of anatomical large intestine. The treatment of the points on this meridian often shows excellent effects.

[3] STOMACH Meridian (ST)

Outline of the Meridian

STOMACH Meridian starts at a deep part of the nose, and comes out below the eye. This meridian consists of two parts. One (chief meridian) goes to the center of the forehead by passing around the mouth, lower jaw, around the face, border of hair. The other one (branch) separating at the middle of the lower jaw, goes down to reach the tip of the 2nd toe via breast, abdomen, inguinal area, and antero-lateral part of the leg.

Details of the Routes

STOMACH Meridian starts at the inside of the nose, and comes to the surface below the eye. After going around the wing of the nose, it enters into the teeth of the upper jaw, and then goes around the mouth, the lower jaw, front of the ear, border of the hair, to reach the center of the border of hairline in the forehead. The branch dividing at the middle of the lower jaw, goes down passing through the anterior part of the neck, center of the supraclavicular fossa (ST_{12}), diaphragm, belonging to STOMACH and connects with SPLEEN. Straight branch goes from ST_{12} via the center of nipple and near the navel to inguinal region ST_{30}. another branch starts at the exit of STOMACH that goes around the inside of abdominal cavity, and reaches ST$_{30}$. There this branch joints with the above mentioned straight branch. Thereafter, the branch goes down passing the antero-lateral part of the upper leg, patella, antero-lateral part of the lower leg, middle part of the foot joint, and the instep of the foot, to reach at the tip of the 2nd toe. Another branch divides from ST$_{36}$ going outside of above mentioned branch, reaches at the tip of the 3rd toe, and the other branch, dividing at the instep, arrives at the 1st toe.

In the general chart, the pathway that goes down from ST$_5$ is regarded as the main pathway of this meridian. According to Reisuu$^{(Jp.)}$ (霊枢), the main pathway runs only in the face. In this book, the pathway from ST$_5$ to ST$_{45}$ is taken as a special branch of the Stomach Meridian.

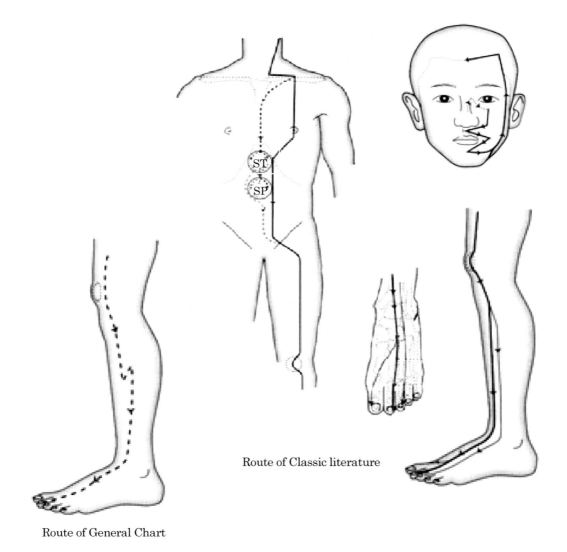

Route of Classic literature

Route of General Chart

Fig.9　STOMACH Meridian

General charts are different from the classic meridian in the following points. General charts are:
1) The meridian starts below the eye, not in the nose.
2) The route from ST_{12} to STOMACH & SPLEEN (principal branch) is not described.
3) The branch from ST_{12} to 2nd toe is regarded as the chief meridian.
4) A branch from the exit of STOMACH to ST_{30} is not described. In many general charts, the branch from ST_{36} to the 3rd toe is not described. The pathway of this part is not always corresponding among general charts.
5) The branch from instep to 1st toe is not described.

STOMACH Meridian and Acupuncture Therapy
Points of STOMACH Meridian are used by following cases with good effects.
1) Treatment of pain of face &/or teeth
2) Treatment of the complaints of the breast
3) Treatment of stomachache
4) Treatment of inguinal region and leg
5) Treatment of the complaints of the nose

Above mentioned cases are complaints of the regions where STOMACH Meridian passes.

6) Treatment of hiccup

According to the FIVE ELEMENT Theory, hiccup is due to disorder of SOIL.
STOMACH and SPLEEN are considered to be the ORGAN of SOIL.
Treatment of hiccup with points of STOMACH Meridian is often astonishingly effective.

[4] SPLEEN Meridian (SP)

Outline of the Meridian
SPLEEN Meridian starts at the 1st toe, and goes up through inside of the leg, inguinal area, abdomen, chest and to under the shoulder joint, where it changes the direction downwards to reach the lateral chest (SP_{21}). Then it turns the direction to upwards, passes the throat, reaches the tongue, and scatters under the tongue.

Details of the routes
SPLEEN Meridian starts at the tibial tip of the 1st toe. It goes along the 1st metatarsus, around the inner ankle, through the inner side of the patella, the antero-median side of the upper leg, inguinal region, belonging to SPLEEN and connects with STOMACH. Then, the meridian goes up through diaphragm to SP_{20} (under the shoulder joint) and it goes down to lateral chest (SP_{21}). From here it goes up again, and passing throat, to reach the root of the tongue and then scatters under the tongue. One branch separates at STOMACH to reach HEART. There are many theories about the pathways of SPLEEN Meridian even among classic literatures.

Mr. SHIROTA Bunshi[3] advocated the existence of three other routes. The first divides from SP_{13} to reach CONCEPTION VESSEL (CV), the second separating from

SP_{15} to reach CV_{10} and the third from SP_{16} to reach CV_{12} belonging to SPLEEN and connecting with STOMACH. These routes are not described in this book.

There are some differences about the route of this meridian around big toe, even among classic literatures. Description of this book follows SAWADA's chart.

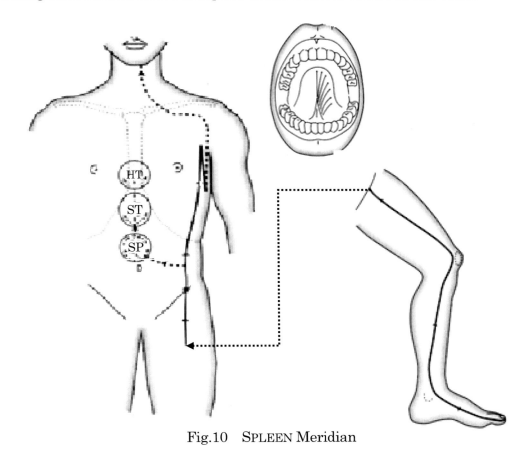

Fig.10 SPLEEN Meridian

General charts are different from the routs of classic literatures as mentioned below. In general charts:
1) The route that enters into abdomen belonging to SPLEEN and connecting with STOMACH is absent
2) The Meridian ends at the lateral chest wall (SP_{21}).
3) The route that goes to the root of the tongue via throat and scatters under the tongue is absent.
4) The route from STOMACH to HEART is absent.
5) The route from SP_{13} to CONCEPTION VESSEL is absent.
6) The route from SP_{15} to CV_{10} is absent.
7) The route from SP_{16} to CV_{12} belonging to SPLEEN and connecting with STOMACH is absent.

SPLEEN Meridian and Acupuncture Therapy
Points of Spleen Meridian are used in the following cases with good effects.
1) Treatment of pain of the legs and the knees (especially pain of inner side).
2) Treatment of pain of the lateral chest.
3) Treatment of pain or abnormal sensation of abdomen.
4) Treatment of complaints in the oral cavity or the tongue,

The above mentioned cases are complaints of the region where SPLEEN Meridian passes. SPLEEN Meridian goes to the tongue through the throat, and scatters under the tongue. For the complaints of the mouth, treatment of this meridian is often very effective.

A classic literature says that there are connections between SPLEEN Meridian and CONCEPTION VESSEL[3]. Referring to this hypothesis, effectiveness of acupuncture of SPLEEN Meridian for the abdominal pain is more easily understandable.

5) Treatment of dysmenorrhea

Most part of the complaint is at the area where SPLEEN Meridian passes. But other complaints such as lumber pain etc. also disappear by the treatment of this meridian. The usually used point for dysmenorrhea is SP_6 or SP_{10}. These points are supposed to have relation with all the IN(Jp.)-meridians of the lower extremity (KIDNEY Meridian and LIVER Meridian). So, this effect may not be due to the effect of only SPLEEN Meridian. Other IN-meridians and CONCEPTION VESSEL may have some participation.

6) Treatment of Impotence

The ORGAN that has influence on reproduction is mostly KIDNEY. LIVER has also some relation with sexual organs. SP_6 and SP_{10} have intimate relation with KIDNEY- and LIVER Meridian. Treatment of these two points is often effective especially for impotence at whiplash syndrome.

7) Treatment of nausea

For the treatment of nausea, usually PERICARDIUM Meridian or LIVER Meridian are used. However, better effect is found by the treatment of Spleen Meridian (especially SP_4). It may be due to "connection with STOMACH".

[5] HEART Meridian (HT)

> **Outline of the Meridian**
> HEART Meridian is consisted of the following three routes
> ① HEART → SMALL INTESTINE
> ② HEART → throat → eye
> ③ HEART → LUNG → under axillary fossa → ulnar side of the arm → tip of the little finger

Details of the routes

HEART Meridian starts from HEART and belongs to HEART System, and goes to SMALL INTESTINE through diaphragm. One branch diverges from HEART System and goes to the eye passing the throat. The main meridian starts from HEART System to LUNG, then goes down to the axillar fossa, and via inner ulnar side of the arm, reaches the radial end of the little finger.

General charts are different from classic meridians as mentioned below.

In the general charts:
1) Meridian from HEART to SMALL INTESTINE (chief meridian) is absent.
2) Meridian to the eye via throat is absent.
3) The route from axillar fossa to little finger (on ③ of mentioned above) is described as chief meridian, and the route from LUNG to axillar fossa is not described.

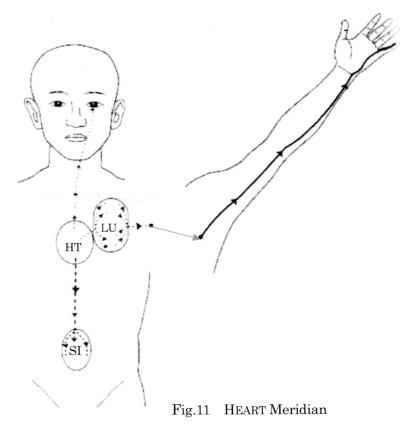

Fig.11   HEART Meridian

HEART Meridian and Acupuncture Therapy

Points of HEART Meridian are used in the following cases with good effects.
1) Treatment of the pain of the upper extremity

HEART Meridian passes through this part. Acupuncture is especially effective for the complaints of the ulnar side.

2) Treatment of the pain due to ischemic heart disease
   According to the classic literatures, HEART Meridian belongs to HEART SYSTEM. Pain caused by ischemic heart disease often appears along the route of HEART Meridian on the arm. Points of HEART Meridian are used according to these facts.
3) Treatment of the complaints of the eye
   In my practice, mainly LIVER Meridian (especially LR$_3$) is used for the complaints of the eye with excellent effect. As HEART Meridian also goes to the eye, sometimes HEART Meridian is used together with LIVER Meridian.
4) Treatment of toss
   As HEART meridian in the classic literatures passes LUNG, sometimes points of HEART Meridian are used together with points of other meridians.

[6] SMALL INTESTINE Meridian

Outline of the Meridian
SMALL INTESTINE Meridian starts from the tip of the little finger, goes along the outer ulnar side of the arm and over the scapula, and reaches supraclavicular fossa. There, it divides into two routes: One goes to HEART and SMALL INTESTINE, and the other goes through the neck and zygomatic area to enter into the ear.

Details of the routes
SMALL INTESTINE Meridian starts from the ulnar end of the small finger, and via outer ulnar side of the arm, goes to the shoulder (on the scapula). After a zigzag course on the scapula, it goes to GV$_{14}$ (middle of C$_7$ and Th$_1$ of the vertebra), and then to supraclavicular fossa (ST$_{12}$) (in Reisuu$^{(Jp.)}$霊枢 [1] this route is not evidently described). From ST$_{12}$, the chief meridian goes down to connect with HEART, then goes around the throat, passes diaphragm, and arrives at SMALL INTESTINE via STOMACH. A branch divides at ST$_{12}$, goes up to lateral neck, zygomatic area, lateral angle of the eye and then into the ear. A branch divides at zygomatic area goes to medial angle of the eye (BL$_1$).

The route in the general charts is almost the same as the route in the classic literatures up to the scapula. Thereafter, however, the route in the general charts deviates widely in the following points. In the general charts:
1) The route that drops by CV$_{14}$ is absent.
2) The chief meridian (throat→HEART→STOMACH→SMALL INTESTINE) is absent.
3) The route passing lateral neck → zygomatic area → ear is describes as the chief meridian. This route directly goes to the zygomatic area without passing ST$_{12}$ and lateral angle of the eye, and it does not enter into the ear.
4) A branch from zygomatic area to medial angle of eye is absent.

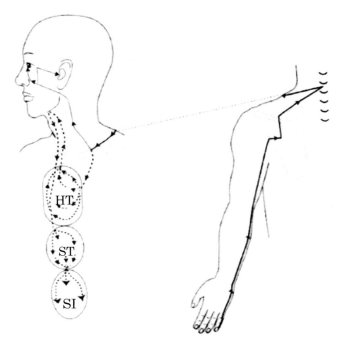

Fig.12　SMALL INTESTINE Meridian

SMALL INTESTINE Meridian and Acupuncture Therapy
　Points of SMALL INTESTINE Meridian are used by following cases with good effects.
1) Treatment of the complaints of the arm
2) Treatment of shoulder stiffness and/or pain (especially around the scapula)
3) Treatment of trigeminal neuralgia (at the area of 2nd branch)
4) Treatment of complaints around the zygomatic area
　The cases 1) to 4) are complaints at where SMALL INTESTINE Meridian passes.
5) Treatment of tinnitus &/or hearing disability
　According to the description of Reisuu$^{(Jp.)}$霊枢 [1] (that this meridian enters into the ear), SMALL INTESTINE Meridian is treated together with other meridians.

[7] BLADDER Meridian (BL)

> **Outline of the Meridian**
> 　BLADDER Meridian starts from the medial angle of the eye, and goes along the pathway parallel to the median line of the head. At around the border of neck and trunk, it divides into two ways. Then they go down the back of the body, and after passing the gluteal region and upper leg, the two ways unify at the popliteal fossa. Thereafter it goes through the posterior center of the lower leg and then the anterior side of Achilles' tendon and reaches the little toe. The meridian has branches at the head and the lower leg.

Details of the Routes

BLADDER Meridian starts from the medial angle of the eye, goes along the pathway parallel to the centerline of the head, and a branch divides at BL7 going to the top of the head (GV$_{20}$) where a branch of GOVERNOR VESSEL (GV) enters into the brain. A branch goes down from GV$_{20}$ goes down the temporal area, and connects with GALLBLADDER Meridian. The chief meridian goes down along the center of the neck, and after going by GV$_{14}$, continues to go down parallel to the median line of the back, relating the distance of about two fingers width from the median line. Around the middle of sacroiliac joint (BL$_{30}$), the meridian goes up and enters into the waist, connects with KIDNEY and belongs to BLADDER.

A branch divides at BL$_{11}$. It goes down in parallel to the outside of the chief meridian at the distance of about two finger width. From the height of BL$_{30}$ (BL$_{54}$), it goes near the grater trochanter, the postero-lateral part of hip joint around the center of sacred bone, gluteal region and back of upper leg, to reach the center of popliteal fossa. Here the two meridians join together, and the united one goes down to the dividing point of gastrocnemius muscle. There the meridian changes the direction to the postero-lateral side of the lower leg, and goes through the front of Achilles' tendon, center of the calcaneus, lateral margin of the foot, to reach the lateral end of the little toe.

Descriptions of the routes of this meridian vary even among the general charts.

(Reisuu$^{(Jp.)}$（霊枢）says that this meridian goes from BL$_7$ → GV$_{20}$ → Brain → BL$_8$ → BL$_9$. Whereas SAWADA's chart says that the main meridian goes BL$_7$ → BL$_8$ → BL$_9$, and a branch goes from BL$_7$ to GV$_{20}$. In this book, SAWADA's chart is given.

In SAWADA's chart, besides the route of GV$_{16}$ → BL$_{10}$ (→ GV$_{14}$), another route from GV$_{16}$ to GV$_{14}$ is given which is not seen in Reisuu（霊枢）. This route is not shown in this book.

There are two parallel BLADDER Meridian routes. Regarding the route of these two routes, SAWADA's chart is shown in this book.

Major differences of the routes between general charts and classic meridian are as described below.

In general charts:
1) BLADDER Meridian does not connect with GOVERNOR VESSEL.
2) Route to the brain (via GV$_{20}$) is absent.
3) The route that connects with GALL BLADDER Meridian at the head is absent.
4) The dividing point of the chief meridian at the back varies.
5) The route that connects with KIDNEY and belongs to BLADDER is not described.
6) The pathways of the routes at the back of the body vary.

BLADDER Meridian and Acupuncture Therapy

Points of Bladder Meridian are used in the following cases with good effects.
1) Treatment of complaints of head &/or nape or shoulder
2) Treatment of back pain

3) Treatment of the lumber pain
4) Treatment of pain of the legs (sciatic neuralgia etc.)
5) Treatment of the knee joint pain
6) Treatment of the ankle joint pain
7) Treatment of the complaints of the nose

   Above mentioned cases are complaints at where BLADDER Meridian passes.

   For the complaints of the nose, points of LARGE INTESTINE Meridian and STOMACH Meridian are mainly used to give an excellent effects. But treatment of the points of BLADDER Meridian are often effective. It may be due to the starting point of BLADDER Meridian, which is situated near the root of the nose

8) Treatment of intercostal neuralgia

   In some cases of intercostal neuralgia of the precordial part or lateral chest or lateral abdomen, the treatment of the points of BLADDER Meridian strongly assists the effect of other meridians. This may be due to the fact that the location of cause of this neuralgia is probably at around the vertebra.

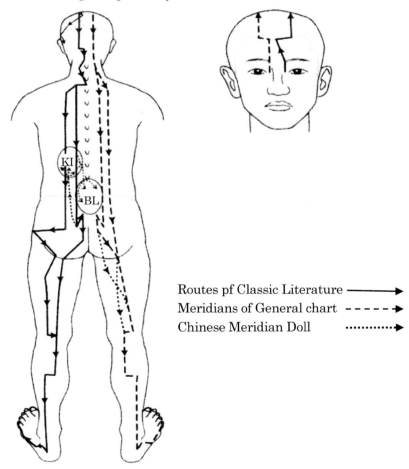

Routes pf Classic Literature ──────▶
Meridians of General chart   ─ ─ ─ ─▶
Chinese Meridian Doll   ·············▶

Fig.13   BLADDER Meridian

[8] KIDNEY Meridian (KI)

Outline of the Meridian
KIDNEY Meridian starts from under the little toe, and goes via center of the sole of foot, the medial side of the heel, and the medial side of the leg to coccygeal region. Then changing the course to abdominal side of the body, it goes up parallel to the centerline of the anterior body to pass through the bronchus, the throat, and then finally reaches the route of the tongue.

Details of the routes
KIDNEY Meridian starts from under the little toe, and going through the center of the sole, under the scaphoid bone, the medial side of the heel, the medial side of the leg (at SP$_6$ it connects with SPLEEN Meridian and LIVER Meridian), arrives at coccygeal region where it connects with GOVERNOR VESSEL (GV). Then the meridian changes the course to abdominal side, to appear at the upper edge of the pubic bone (KI$_{11}$). Thereafter it goes up in parallel to the ventral center line of the body (width of one or half a thumb apart from the centerline of the body). The meridian connects with KIDNEY at the height of the navel, then goes down and connects with BLADDER. The other meridian passes LIVER and diaphragm, goes up to LUNG, and arrives at the root of the tongue (end of CONCEPTION VESSEL) via the bronchus and throat. A branch divides from LUNG, which connects with HEART and flows into the chest.

Marked differences are seen in the pathway and points of KIDNEY Meridian between different literatures, especially in the route between KI$_2$ and KI$_7$.

In general charts, the pathway is shown: KI$_2$ → KI$_3$ → KI$_4$ → KI$_5$ → KI$_6$ → KI$_7$, drawing a loop. There are another type of the route which does not make loop-shaped pathway (SAWADA's chart or Ruikei-zuyoku$^{(Jp.)}$ 類経図翼(Illustrated Appendices to the Categories). According to my experience of acupoint injection, the route of general charts seems more reasonable. In PART1 Chapter 4 § 3 of this book, both, general charts and SAWADA's chart, are given. As regards the pathway of this meridian and location of points, there are many different opinions. This may be due to individual difference of human body. But I cannot abandon the idea that the shape of KIDNEY Meridian is not linear but band shaped in this area.

General charts are different from classic chart as described below.

In general charts:
1) The meridian starts from the center of the sole.
2) The chief meridian ends at around the medial end of the clavicle, and the route to the throat and the tongue is absent.
3) The route that connects with KIDNEY and BLADDER is absent.
4) A branch starting from LUNG, going to HEART, and flows into the chest is absent.

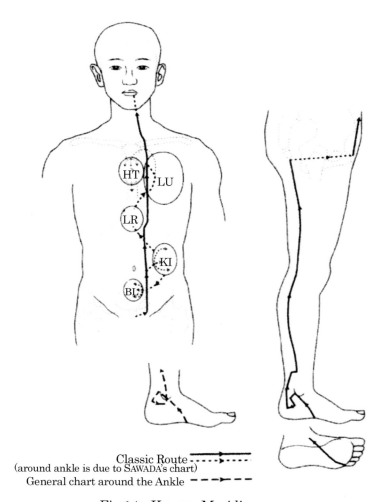

Classic Route
(around ankle is due to SAWADA's chart)
General chart around the Ankle

Fig.14 KIDNEY Meridian

KIDNEY Meridian and Acupuncture Therapy

In my practice, the most basic principle of meridian selection is to select meridians that pass the place of complaints. KIDNEY Meridian is often selected on the different principles.

Points of KIDNEY Meridian are used in the following cases.

1) Treatment of the complaints at the medial and back side of leg and the complaints at the abdomen or the anterior chest
2) Treatment of pain around anus

   CV_{20} is mostly used for the anal pain treatment. However, as the anal region is near to the coccygeal bone, the points of KIDNEY Meridian are often tried for anal pain with fairly good effect.

3) Treatment of bronchial asthma

Many patients with asthmatic attack suffer from strong discomfort at sternal region &/or throat where KIDNEY Meridian passes. According to the classic literatures, KIDNEY Meridian enters into LUNG. Furthermore, Oriental Medicine regards asthma as the disorder of WATER. KIDNEY is the ORGAN that controls WATER. Thus the treatment of KIDNEY Meridian for bronchial asthma may be quite reasonable. Actually, it always gives excellent effects.

Relation among KIDNEY and immunity and allergy will be explained later.

4) Treatment of pain or abnormal sensation of the throat
5) Treatment of hoarseness
6) Treatment of dysphagia

4)〜6) is based on the classic literatures which says that KIDNEY Meridian passes through throat and arrives at the root of the tongue. Sometimes auricular acupuncture is also performed along with body acupuncture.

7) Treatment of the urogenital organs

According to the classic literatures, this meridian connects with KIDNEY and BLADDER. The points on KIDNEY Meridian are used for the treatment of pain or urinal disorders due to diseases of prostate, cystitis or dysmenorrhea. They are often used along with SPLEEN Meridian &/or LIVER Meridian.

8) Treatment of tinnitus or vertigo

Classic literature says "KIDNEY controls the Ear.", and that these symptoms are due to disorder of WATER. Following based on this concept, points of KIDNEY Meridian are used even though this meridian does not pass the ear. Often this meridian is used along with other meridians &/or auricular acupuncture.

9) Treatment of disorders of the bone

Classic literature says "KIDNEY controls bone". Accordingly, points of KIDNEY Meridian are used for the treatment of disorders related to the bone disease in my practice.

10) Treatment of allergic disease (This will be mentioned in PART6 §12).

I do not believe that KIDNEY and kidney are the same. According to the description of classic literatures, function of KIDNEY is almost the same as that of the system of hypothalamus-adrenal body-gonads, especially adrenal body. In that sense, in my practice, the points on KIDNEY Meridian are always used for allergic diseases or autoimmune disease for which steroid hormones are used, and excellent effects are always obtained. The effect for bronchial asthma may contain this factor. For the disorders of the joint, the points on KIDNEY Meridian are used in the same reason.

[9] PERICARDIUM Meridian (PC)

> **Outline of the Meridian**
> PERICARDIUM Meridian starts in the thorax, and from PERICARDIUM it goes around the UPPER-, MIDDLE- and LOWER- ENERGIZER. A branch that starts from PERICARDIUM appears at the anterior chest, and reaches at the tip of the middle finger.

Details of the routes

PERICARDIUM Meridian, belonging to PERICARDIUM, starts in the thorax. It goes down through the diaphragm, and goes around UPPER ENERGIZER, MIDDLE ENERGIZER and LOWER ENERGIZER. A branch, after going around inside of the chest, appears at the anterior chest, and goes along the center line of flexor side of arm to reach the radial end of middle finger. One branch divides at the center of palm which goes to the ring finger connecting with TRIPLE ENERGIZER Meridian.

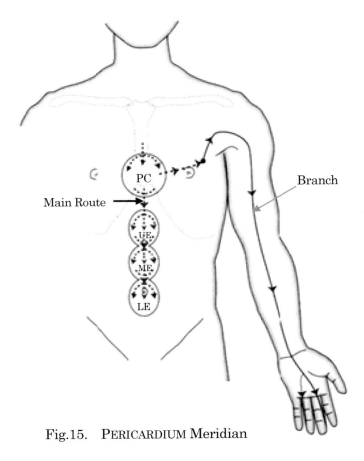

Fig.15. PERICARDIUM Meridian

General charts are different from the classic literature as described below.
In general charts:
1) Chief meridian is completely absent.
2) A part of the branch (inside of the chest to anterior chest) is not described, and the route from the anterior chest to the tip of middle finger is described as the chief meridian.
3) A branch from the palm to the ring finger is absent.

PERICARDIUM Meridian and Acupuncture Therapy
Points of PERICARDIUM Meridian are used in the following cases.
1) Treatment of the pain at the flexor side of arm, axillar fossa and anterior chest.
2) Treatment of the pain of the shoulder joint

These cases are complaints at the places where PERICARDIUM Meridian passes.
3) Treatment of palpitation and pain caused by cardiac vascular diseases
4) Treatment of pain of cardiac disease

Pain due to cardiac vascular disease often appears along the pathway of this meridian. PC_5 and PC_6 are closely related with LUNG Meridian & HEART Meridian. The use 3) and 4) is according to the facts mentioned above.

5) Treatment of myasthenia gravis

There is no anatomic organ corresponding to "PERICARDIUM". According to the description of the classic literatures, PERICARDIUM is situated at CV_{17} (at about the middle of the sternum) near (in front of?) HEART, and it has a network[8]. Thus, the location and the form of PERICARDIUM are quite similar to those of thymus. Considering the situation and the fact that thymectomy is often effective for myasthenia gravis, treatment of PC_5 was tried with the points of other meridians. Apparently it was effective to a certain extent, especially for the disorder of the eye such as eyelid ptosis or diplopia.

6) Treatment of allergic diseases (This will be mentioned in PART6 §12.)

Thymus has close relation to immunity. In my practice, since PERICARDIUM has an obvious resemblance to thymus, points on PERICARDIUM Meridian (usually PC_5) are principally used together with points on KIDNEY Meridian for the treatment of allergic diseases or autoimmune diseases.

[10] TRIPLE ENERGIZER Meridian (TE)

Outline of the Meridian
TRIPLE ENERGIZER Meridian starts from the tip of the ring finger, and going along the dorsum of the hand, the median line of the arm (extensor side) and around the upper part of the scapula, and arrives at the supraclavicular fossa (ST_{12}). Thereafter it goes down into the chest and reach PERICARDIUM and TRIPLE ENERGIZER. A branch divides in the chest, and reappears at the supraclavicular fossa. Then it goes to the temporal region via lateral neck and retro-auricular region taking complicated pathways.

Details of the Routes

TRIPLE ENERGIZER Meridian starts from the ulnar end of ring finger. The route is: origin → between the 4th and 5th metacarpus → center of the extensor side of hand joint → median line of the arm → acromion of scapula → near the margin of the scapula → supraclavicular fossa (ST$_{12}$). Hereafter, it goes down into the chest and connects with PERICARDIUM at CV$_{17}$. Then, passing through the diaphragm, it belongs to TRIPLE ENERGIZER. According to the classic literature[3], it connects with UPPER ENERGIZER at around the entrance of STOMACH, then with MIDDLE ENERGIZER at CV$_{12}$, and finally with LOWER ENERGIZER at CV$_7$. A branch separating at CV$_{17}$ goes up and reappears at ST$_{12}$, after stopping by GV$_{14}$ (in Reisuu$^{(Jp.)}$霊枢 this description is absent), the meridian goes via the retro-auricular region and the cheek, to reach the zygomatic bone. A branch dividing from TE$_{17}$ (under the auricle) enters into the ear, reappears at SI$_{19}$ and passing the anterior part of GB$_3$, arrives at the lateral angle of the eye.

As regards the pathway in the face, there are various views even among the classic literatures.

General charts are different from classic literatures as described below.

In general charts:

1) The route is drawn as "from TE$_{15}$ to posterior part of the neck and posterior part of the auricle". Thus, the route to PERICARDIUM and TRIPLE ENERGIZER (chief meridian) is absent.
2) A part of the branch that reappears at ST$_{12}$ from CV$_{17}$ is regarded as the chief meridian, and here, the description of general chart is extremely different from that of classic literatures as described below:
   ① The route CV$_{17}$ → supraclavicular fossa → GV$_{14}$ → lateral neck is absent.
   ② The route TE$_{17}$ → enters into the ear is absent.
   ③ The route TE$_{17}$ → retro-auricular part → forehead → medial angle of eye → zygomatic bone is absent.
   ④ Instead of route ③, route ② goes directly from the upper part of the tragus (TE$_{21}$) to TE$_{23}$, not passing GB$_1$.

TRIPLE ENERGIZER Meridian and Acupuncture Therapy

Points of TRIPLE ENERGIZER Meridian are used by following cases.

1) Treatment of headache (especially at temple)
2) Treatment of shoulder stiffness and pain of the neck
3) Treatment of complaint of the shoulder joint
4) Treatment of pain or numbness of the arm.
   These cases are for the complaints located at where TRIPLE ENERGIZER Meridian passes.
5) Treatment of tinnitus &/or dizziness
   According to the classic literature that this meridian enters into the ear.

6) Treatment of complaints of forehead
According to a classic literature[3] this meridian passes forehead.

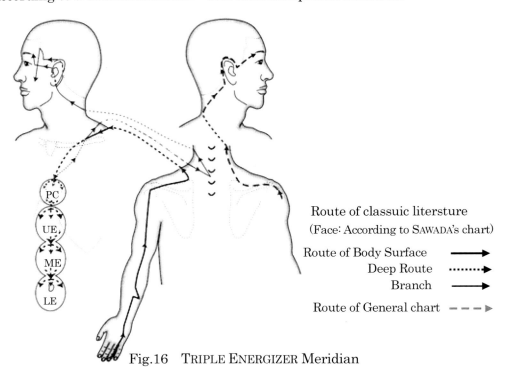

Fig.16 TRIPLE ENERGIZER Meridian

[11] GALLBLADDER Meridian (GB)

Outline of the Meridian
GALLBLADDER Meridian starts at the lateral angle of the eye, and passing quite complicated pathways through the face and head, reaches the nape of the neck. Thereafter, going through the shoulder → the anterior-lateral chest → the lateral abdomen → the greater trochanter → the lateral side of the leg, to reach the tip of the 4th toe.

Details of the routes
GALLBLADDER Meridian has many branches, and connects with many other meridians. The pathway of this meridian is quite complicated and even among the classic literatures the description is not always the same. Thus, it is quite difficult to understand its routes.

According to SAWADA's chart[3] GALLBLADDER Meridian arises from lateral angle of the eye (GB_1), passes very complicated pathway of the face and the head, and via GV_{14}, BL_{11}, SI_{12} and shoulder, reaches supraclavicular fossa (ST_{12}). Then it goes down refracting on the lateral & anterior chest and abdomen, reaches near the grater trochanter, and goes down along the center of the lateral side of the leg and between the 4th and 5th metatarsal bone, arrives at the fibular tip of the 4th toe.

A branch divides at occipital region (GB$_{20}$) and enters into the ear. A branch divides from GB$_1$ reaches below eye via ST$_5$. A branch divides from ST$_5$, enters into the chest via ST$_{12}$, and passing through chest, connecting with LIVER and GALLBLADDER, it goes to inguinal region (ST$_{30}$) and arrives at GB$_{30}$. A branch divides from GB$_{41}$, and goes to LR$_1$ connecting with LIVER Meridian.

About the routes of GALLBLADDER Meridian, there are different theories even among classic literatures. For example, SAWADA's chart[3] shows the route TE$_{20}$ → GB$_{13}$ → BL$_4$ → GB$_{14}$ → BL$_1$ → GB$_{15}$, whereas there is no such route is shown in Reisuu[1]. (In this book, the route of Sawada's chart is shown, because I have many experiences of acupoint injection by which wide range complaints of forehead were alleviated by injection at GB$_{41}$, GB$_{42}$ or GB$_{43}$.)

In general chart, the location of GB$_{35}$ is illustrated posterior to GB$_{36}$. In Sawada's chart, GB$_{35}$ is illustrated anterior to GB$_{36}$. In this book, the route of general chart is shown.

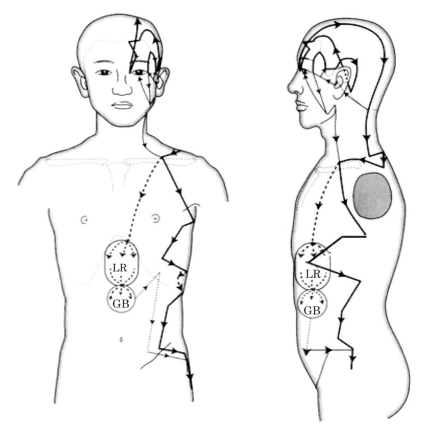

Fig.17-1 GALLBLADDER Meridian (Head, Face and Trunk)

36 PART 1 INTRODUCTION — OUTLINE OF ACUPUNCTURE —

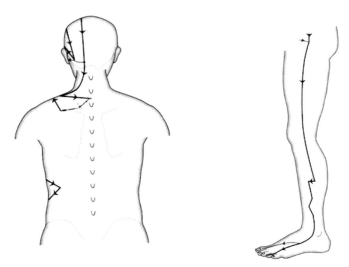

Fig.17-2 GALLBLADDER Meridian (Neck, Back of Trunk and Leg)

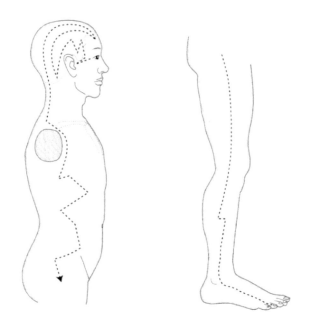

Fig.18 GALLBLADDER Meridian (General Chart)

　The route of general chart is very simple, different from routes of classic literature as described below.
1) The route of general charts has no connection with other meridians.
2) The route at head and face is remarkably simplified and it has no branch.
3) The branch from GB_1 → ST_5 → below the eye is absent.
4) The branch from GB_{20} to ear is absent.

5) Chief meridian does not go to ST_{12}, and passes the anterior side of the shoulder joint.
6) The branch from ST_5 → ST_{12} → into the chest → connecting with GALLBLADDER and LIVER → ST_{30} → GB_{30} is absent.
7) The branch from GB_{41} to LR_1 is absent.

The route of general chart is quite simplified and different from routes of classic literature as Fig.18.

GALLBLADDER Meridian and Acupuncture Therapy
Treatment of GALLBLADDER Meridian is used by following cases.
1) Treatment of headache
2) Treatment of pain &/or stiffness of neck and shoulder
3) Treatment of chest pain
4) Treatment of pain of the leg

These are for complaints located at where GALLBLADDER Meridian passes.

5) Treatment of lumbar pain

Patient with lumbar pain mostly have pain at the region where BLADDER Meridian passes, and mainly points of BLADDER Meridian are used for the treatment of lumber pain. However, some patients complain pain at lateral abdominal part. Some classic literatures say that this meridian goes from sacral region to coccygeal region. And the point GB_{26} is on the extra meridian "BELT VESSEL" which passes around L_3 of the vertebra. In these meanings, points of GALLBLADDER Meridian are used for almost all the patients of lumbar pain. It seems more effective than the treatment of BLADDER Meridian alone.

6) Treatment of complaints of the eye

Classic literature[1] says that this meridian goes to eye. In my practice, usually points of LIVER Meridian is used for the complaints of the eye. But treatment of points of GALLBLADDER Meridian is sometimes very effective.

7) Treatment of tinnitus, vertigo or deafness

Considering classic literature's description[1] that GALLBLADDER Meridian enters into the ear, points of this meridian are used together with KIDNEY Meridian and TRIPLE ENERGIZER Meridian. Incidentally, according to FIVE ELEMENT Theory, dizziness is disturbance of WOOD, and GALLBLADDER is an ORGAN of WOOD. Points of GALLBLADDER Meridian are used for dizziness considering this theory and it is often very effective.

[12] LIVER Meridian (LR)

> **Outline of the Meridian**
> LIVER Meridian starts from big toe. It goes along dorsum of the foot, and then → around external genitalia → the lower abdomen → the lateral abdomen → the throat → the eye and reaches the top of the head (GV_{20}).

Details of the routes

LIVER Meridian starts from the root of nail (fibular side) of the big toe, and goes between 1st and 2nd metatarsus → medial side of the leg → around external genitalia → lower abdomen. (According to SAWADA's chart, from here it goes up with CONCEPTION VESSEL to STOMACH, belongs to LIVER and connects with GALLBLADDER). Then it passes through diaphragm, distributes in the lateral chest wall, goes up along trachea, passes the throat, eye, forehead, and arrives at the top of the head (GV$_{20}$). A branch divides from the eye and goes to the lip passing inside of the cheek. One branch divides from LIVER, penetrates the diaphragm, goes to LUNG and connects with LUNG.

(This meridian has branches reaching ORGANs of inner part of the body. Although its line is drawn on the surface of body in many charts, its real pathway of the body may be difficult to identify. So, the route of this meridian is drawn as a schema in this book.)

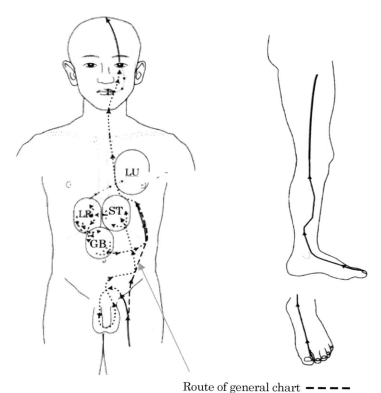

Route of general chart ----

Fig.19　LIVER Meridian

General charts are different from classic literatures as described below.
1) In some general charts LIVER Meridian does not pass external genitalia.
2) Neither the route which goes → STOMACH → LIVER → GALLBLADDER nor the route (as SAWADA's chart) which goes up with CONCEPTION VESSEL is described,

and the meridian is illustrated simply from medial side of leg to lateral side of lower chest (to go LR$_{14}$).
3) The meridian stops at the chest. Therefor:
① The route which passes along trachea and throat is absent.
② The meridian does not pass the eye, and it does not reach GV$_{20}$.
③ The branch which goes to lip passing inside of the cheek is absent.
4) The route from LIVER to LUNG is absent.

LIVER Meridian and Acupuncture Therapy

Treatment of LIVER Meridian is used by following cases.
1) Treatment of pain of the leg and the knee joint.
2) Treatment of abdominal pain.
   These cases are complaints located at where LIVER Meridian passes.
3) Treatment of disorders of genital organs
   According to the description of classic literatures LIVER Meridian goes around the external genitalia. Points of LIVER Meridian are used with KIDNEY Meridian.
4) Treatment of disorders of the eye
5) Treatment of disorders of the mouth &/or lip
   The reason of meridian selection of 4) and 5) is the routes of classic literatures.
6) Treatment of anal pain
   For the disorders of the anal region, GV$_{20}$ is often treated. Considering that LIVER Meridian goes to GV$_{20}$, LR$_3$ was tried to use with KIDNEY Meridian, and it is often effective.

[13] GOVERNOR VESSEL (GV)

> **Outline of the Meridian**
> Governor Vessel arises in lower abdomen, after going around the external genitalia goes to the perineum, and goes up along the median line of the back and head, and arrives at upper lip.

Details of the Routes

GOVERNOR VESSEL is not described in Reisuu[(Jp.)1]. According to the description of Somon[(Jp.)2], GOVERNOR VESSEL arises in the lower abdomen, goes down to the pubic symphysis, going around external genitalia, arrives at the perineum. Chief meridian starts from here, and goes up along the median line of the back, neck and head, and arrives at upper lip. The other meridian goes around the gluteal region, and enters into KIDNEY with KIDNEY Meridian. The other meridian arises from the medial angle of the eye (BL$_1$), goes up to the top of the head, enters into the brain, and after connecting with brain, reappears and goes down along vertebra, and enters into KIDNEY. Other meridian goes up from the lower abdomen, through navel and HEART, passes throat and around lip and arrives at the lower eyelid. This meridian seems closely resembles CONCEPTION Vessel (CV).

General chart describes only one route, from perineum to upper lip.

The description of Somon(Jp.)2) is different from general charts as described below.

1) GOVERNOR VESSEL of Somon(Jp.)2) contains pleural meridians and it seems a complex of meridians.
2) GOVERNOR VESSEL has a route from the lower abdomen to KIDNEY.
3) GOVERNOR VESSEL has a route that connects with KIDNEY together with BLADDER Meridian and KIDNEY Meridian.
4) The route from BL_1 to GV_{20} (same as BLADDER Meridian) is described as GOVERNOR VESSEL.
5) GOVERNOR VESSEL has a route from GV_{20} to lumber region and enters into KIDNEY.
6) A route that goes up the abdomen (very similar to CONCEPTION VESSEL) is described as GOVERNOR VESSEL.

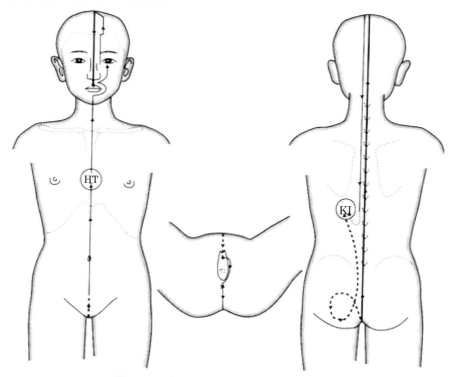

Fig.20　GOVERNOR VESSEL
(General chart shows only the route from perineum to upper lip.)

GOVERNOR VESSEL and Acupuncture Therapy

It is ssaid that GOVERNOR VESSEL is an important meridian which unify YO-U(Jp.)(YANG(Ch.)) meridians (LI, ST, SI, BL, TE & GB), and all the points of this meridian are very important. Generally, points of this meridian are widely used as stream points of BLADDER Meridian. But it seems that almost all the indications of this meridian can be substituted by the points of BLADDER Meridian. So, in my practice, the points of GOVERNOR VESSEL are scarcely used except GV_{14}.

GOVERNOR VESSEL is used for the treatment of following cases.

1) Treatment of pain along the median line of head and trunk.

Points of this meridian are used when the treatment of BLADDER Meridian is not enough effective, but it is rather rare.

2) Auxiliary use of treatment of the complaints of shoulder &/or arm.

When the treatment of shoulder or arm is not enough effective, acupoint injection to GV_{14} is often added. It is very useful.

3) Treatment of hemorrhoid

Moxibustion at GV_{20} is often used for the treatment of hemorrhoid. Since this part is usually covered with hair, it is inconvenient to use because of difficulty of disinfection.

4) Treatment of hangover

GV_{20} is used for hangover. This is an oral instruction of the late Dr. MANAKA. Retaining needle or acupoint injection is sometimes fairly effective.

5) According to the description of classis literature, all the YO-U[Jp.] meridians except Stomach Meridian converge on GV_{14}. Acupoint injection to GV_{14} often causes excellent effect for wide spread complaints.

[14] CONCEPTION VESSEL (CV)

> **Outline of the Meridian**
> CONCEPTION VESSEL arises from the lesser pelvis, and passing perineum, goes up along the anterior median line, and through the throat and the chin, goes around lip, and enters into the eye.

Details of the Routes

Reisuu[Jp.)1] says that "CONCEPTION VESSEL arises in the uterus (?), and goes around the retroperitoneal region (?). Other route goes out and goes up to the throat and goes around the lip and the mouth." Somon[Jp.)2] says "CONCEPTION VESSEL arises under CV_3, goes up to the edge of pubes, goes around inner side of the abdomen, goes up to CV_4 and goes up to → the throat → the chin → and around face, and enters into the eye." "Under CV_3" may mean the uterus. Namely, CONCEPTION VESSEL can be regarded to arise from the lesser pelvis, and the route is → the perineum → along the median line of the abdomen → center of the chin → angle of the mouth → center of the upper mouth (here it connects with GOVERNOR VESSEL) → outer side of the wing of nose → the eye. As is mentioned above, one route of GOVERNOR VESSEL is described as very similar route.

42   PART 1   INTRODUCTION – OUTLINE OF ACUPUNCTURE –

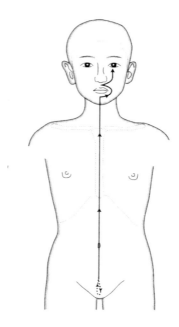

Fig.21   CONCEPTION VESSEL
(General chart shows only the route from perineum to lower lip)

General chart is different from classic literature as described below.
In general chart:
1) The meridian arises from perineum.
2) The route ends at the center of lower lip, and the route to eye is absent.
CONCEPTION VESSEL and Acupuncture Therapy
It is said that CONCEPTION VESSEL is an important meridian which unify IN$^{(Jp.)}$ (YIN$^{(Ch.)}$) meridians (LU, SP, HT, KI, PC, & LR), and all the points on this meridian are very important. Generally, points of this meridian are widely used. However, in my practice, almost all these cases can be treated using points on ST, SP, KI, &/or LR Meridians. And also, the point of this meridian is used for the complaints of medial region of chest and abdomen only when the effect is unsatisfying, and sometimes for the complaints of the eye (with acupoint injection).

[15] Important Meridians That are not Described in Usual Charts

General charts are described simplified, and almost all the branches are not described except STOMACH Meridian and BLADDER Meridian. But there are not few cases which classic meridians are inevitable. Among hidden meridians not described in general charts, followings are important in my practice.
LU: The meridian connects LARGE INTESTINE and belongs to LUNG.
   Skin and hair belong to LUNG.

LI: The meridian connects with LUNG and belongs to LARGE INTESTINE.
   The meridian passes teeth of the lower jaw.
ST: The meridian starts from the inner nose.
   The meridian belongs to SPLEEN and connects with STOMACH.
SP: The meridian belongs to SPLEEN and connects with STOMACH.
   The meridian passes throat and spreads under the tongue.
HT: The meridian belongs to HEART and connects with SMALL INTESTINE.
   The meridian passes the throat and goes to the eye system.
   A route goes from HEART to LUNG.
SI: The meridian connects with HEART, goes around the throat, and through STOMACH belongs to SMALL INTESTINE.
   The meridian enters into the ear.
BL: The meridian goes to GV_{20} and connects with the brain.
   The meridian connects with KIDNEY and belongs to Bladder.
KI: The meridian belongs to KIDNEY and connects with BLADDER.
   Chief route is KIDNEY → LIVER → LUNG → Throat → Tongue
   A branch leaves LUNG, connects with HEART and goes into the chest.
PC: The meridian belongs to PERICARDIUM and connects with TRIPLE ENERGIZER
   A route goes around in the chest.
TE: The meridian goes to PERICARDIUM and belongs to TRIPLE ENERGIZER.
   A branch passes the forehead, and the other goes from medial angle of eye to zygomatic area.
   A branch goes into the ear.
GB: The meridian connects with many meridians (ST, SI, BL, TE, & GV).
   A branch enters the ear.
   A branch goes to the eye.
   The route passes the forehead.
   The meridian goes down through the chest and connects with LIVER, and belongs to GALLBLADDER.
LR: The meridian passes the external genitalia.
   The meridian connects with Liver, GALLBLADDER and STOMACH.
   The meridian passes the throat and eye.
   The meridian appears at the forehead and goes to the top of the head.
   A branch passes the cheek and goes around the lip.
   A branch enters LUNG.
GV: All YO-U[Jp.] (YANG[Ch.]) Meridians except STOMACH Meridian pass GV_{14}.
CV: It goes around the lip, and enters into the eye.

§ 4 Acupuncture Point (Acupoint)

[1] What is Acupuncture Point?

"Toothache suddenly reduced by applying finger pressure at a point between the thumb and the index finger!"

That kind of experiences may not be rare. Like this case, there are points that cause some reaction in the body by some stimulation. Such points are called "acupuncture point" or "acupoint" or simply "point" (in Japanese "Tsubo"). Each point is well known to have close relation with certain part of the body. By connecting points with similar character, a line is drawn on the surface of the skin. The concept "meridian" must be formed by the insight into such phenomena. Certainly, acupuncture points are not only the window of organs but also the window of meridians.

Strategy of point selection for treatment is quite different by each school, and by each practitioner. If a beginner wants to investigate a point for some disease, the more he read books, the more he will be confused.

There are many hypotheses about the structure of the point, but theory about it has not been established yet. There is no doubt that acupuncture points actually exist. Points may have some construction. But I have some doubt if acupuncture point would have definite structure, because point seems to move.

In ancient China, there was "Copper-man (Fig.22)". It is a doll made of copper punched small pits at the acupuncture points. It was used by qualifying examination of acupuncturist, being covered with wax and filled with water inside. That must be on the promise that acupuncture points are immobile.

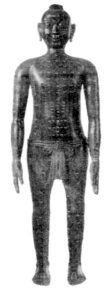

Fig.22   Copper-man
(Photographed by the author at Palace Museum in Beijing)

On the other hand, there is Japanese saying "Sanri sara hitotsu". "Sanri" is ST_{36}, "sara" is dish (here it means patella) "hitotsu" is one. Namely, this phrase means that the location of Leg-SanriST_{36} is not definite but it is situated (or moves) in the range of size of patella. There is a difference of opinion if the position of points is fixed or not. But many professional acupuncturists actually feel that position of acupuncture points is not fixed but varies subtly by person to person, every other time. Someone says that "point of fishing" is not only different for each fish, but not the same according to weather or condition of tide, even for the same fish. Assuming that acupuncture point has both morphological and functional aspects, this phenomenon may be easily understood.

It is said that international agreement of the position of acupuncture point is groped under the leadership of WHO. But, as it will be mentioned later, there is individual difference in the position of acupuncture points, and even in the same person, the position is not always constant. Therefore, it may become irrelevant when the position of points are rigidly followed to the description of textbook. The position of points in meridian chart is better to be regarded as rough standard.

Meridians (and acupuncture points) have connection with ORGANs? or organs? ORGANs of Oriental Medicine and organ of Occidental Medicine are evidently not the same. But acupuncture influences both ORGAN and organ. So, it may be better to take this phenomenon that meridians (and acupuncture points) are connected with both morphological organs and functional ORGANs.

[2] **Name of Points and Their Notation** (c.f. p ix)

In a classic literature of about 2000years ago, 138 names of points are described. After various transitions, about 1000 years ago, present 361 names are established[9]

As acupuncture therapy extends out of Chinese letter area, translated naming appeared in each region, and same point became to bear various names. The People's Republic China proposed to unify the name into modern Chinese name. But no matter who thinks over, it is quite unreasonable. First of all, Chinese Roman transcription (Ping-in), as well as pronunciation and accent, is extremely difficult. Probably nobody, except Chinese, can read "Hegu（合谷）" as "huukuuu", and this pronunciation is also completely different from Chinese itself.

WHO made plan to enact universal name of acupuncture points. Tentative plan was agreed, for the moment, in 1982 at the conference in Manila, and finally it was decided in 1989 at the conference in Geneva.

That is: as the name of meridians, two letters are chosen from the English name of meridian written in capital letters, and after the meridian name, number of points which are given following the order of the meridian's flow. (STOMACH Meridian and BLADDER Meridian are exceptional because they have two lines). Thus the points are quite obvious by this code number. In this book, names of points are always shown by this WHO code number (code name).

[3] Frequently Used Points and Their Location

Here, frequently used points **in my practice** and important standard points for locating points are described.

In my practice, points are used mainly at the peripheral part of extremities, namely distal from the elbow joint and the knee joint. The reason is that the points of other parts are inconvenient to use because of following conditions.

1) Head is usually covered with hair. It is inconvenient for disinfection..
2) Face has rich vascularization, and bleeding occurs easily. The risk and effect of bleeding and making bruise is not negligible.
3) In the region of the neck, there are many important organs, nerves and vessels. So it is hesitated to insert needle at the neck.
4) At the chest wall and the supraclavicular fossa, risk of pneumothorax by needle puncture is not negligible.
5) For the use of points of trunk, it is inevitable to take off clothes. It is not so easy because of the problem of shame, and room heating is indispensable in winter. Time consuming by desorption of clothes is not negligible.

Using points of extremities, especially distal from the elbow and the knee joints, above mentioned inconvenience can be completely prevented. In my field of acupuncture therapy, by the treatment of points only at this area, excellent effects are almost always obtained. So the necessity to use above mentioned inconvenient points is not felt. Main exception is by case of sensory paralysis. Acupuncture treatment at the sensory paralyzed region is ineffective with any method of acupuncture. In such cases, the points at head or trunk must be used.

There are several methods to seek points. But, here, position of points is indicated by "Bone Procportional Cun" which is the standard method named by WHO.

A. Bone Proportional Cun$^{(Ch)}$※. (abbreviation B-cun) (尺度法 **Shakudohou**$^{(Jp.)}$)

This is a method to determine the place of a point by the distance from the anatomical landmarks. The unit of length is put "Sun $^{(Jp.)}$ (Cun$^{(Ch.)}$)" and "Shaku$^{(Jp.)}$ (Chi$^{(Ch.)}$) ".

$1\ \text{Shaku}^{(Jp.)} = 10\ \text{Sun}^{(Jp.)} = 100\ \text{Bu}^{(Jp.)}\ (\fallingdotseq 30.3\text{cm})$.

But this measure is not official unit of absolute length but a variable measure of the individual body. So, the effective value of the length of Shaku$^{(Jp.)}$ or Sun$^{(Jp.)}$ is different by the size of the patient.

That is as described below:

  Height of the patient: 7.5 Shaku$^{(Jp.)}$ (= 7shaku 5sun)
   (As if the patient is a baby.)
  Chest size: 2.6 Shaku (= 2 Shaku 6 Sun)
  Medial malleolus of Tibia — ground: 3 Sun
  Popliteal region — calcaneal tubercle: 1.6 Shaku$^{(Jp.)}$
  Hip Joint — Knee: 1.9 Shaku
  Knee — Lateral Malleolus: 1.6 Shaku
  Between two nipples: 9 Sun

   ※Pronunciation is "tsun"

Length of the foot: 1.2 Shaku
Width of foot: 4.5 Sun (= 4 Sun 5 Bu)
Shoulder — Elbow: 1.2 Shaku
Elbow — Hand Joint: 1.2 Shaku
Hand Joint — MPJ of Middle Finger: 4 Sun
MPJ of Middle Finger — Tip of the Finger: 4.5 Sun   etc.

As practical barometer, width of the thumb = 1Sun, the middle phalanx of middle finger = 1 Sun and width of four fingers (index finger — little finger) = 3 Sun are convenient (Fig.23).

This measurement can be applied for everyone, regardless of the size of the body. But this standard is not precise. Everybody will easily understand it, testing it by the own body. To begin with, the definition of exact location of the standard point is uncertain. But, as mentioned before, the position of point is personally different and it is not always fixed. The position of the points on the meridian chart may be better to be regarded as a rough standard, and this method is very convenient to use. In some books, the place of the points is indicated in cm (instead of Sun) from the standard points. But it may be rather practically incorrect. In some books, the position of points is indicated by proportion between standard points (thereafter this type of indication is called "proportion method"). This method is also very practical.

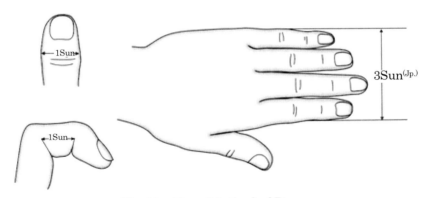

Fig.23   Easy Method of B-cun

B. Points of Each Meridian

Here the aspects of the points are described that are used frequently in my practice, such as names of the points (WHO Code), (the names in correct Chinese letters), their names in English, their position, attentions by the use and the aim of the use of points. The position of points are described according to the SAWADA's chart[3] by B-cun. Description of proportion method is according to the chart of Mr. KINOSHITA Haruto[9] (hereafter this chart is called KINOSHITA's chart). Between SAWADA's chart and KINOSHITA's chart, the positions of points are not always the

48   PART 1 INTRODUCTION – OUTLINE OF ACUPUNCTURE –

same, and there are also various other opinions about the position. But, from the standpoint of view that the position of points should be regarded to be rough standard, the difference may be negligible

1. Points of LUNG Meridian (LU) (Fig.24)

LU$_5$ (尺澤) : Ch'ih-Tze, Short-narrow marsh

This point is situated on the flexor side line of the elbow joint, 0.5 Sun$^{(Jp.)}$ (about the nail of the little finger breadth) from the radial end of the line. This point is important as the standard point of B-cun.

LU$_9$ (太淵) : Tai-Yuen, Great gulf

This point is situated on the line of the hand joint, above the radial artery. This point is important as the standard point of. B-cun

LU$_6$ (孔最) : K'ung-Tzuei, Supreme cave

This point is situated on the line between LU$_5$ and LU$_9$, 7Sun (Cun$^{(Ch.)}$) from LU$_5$, 5.5 Sun(Cun) from LU$_9$, at 2/5 near LU$_5$. This point is most convenient for moxa needle treatment.

LU$_7$ (列缺) : Lieh-Ch'üeh, Extreme shortcoming

This point is situated on the line between LU$_5$ and LU$_9$, 2.5 Sun(Cun) (about 2 fb.) from LU$_9$, at 1/8 near LU$_9$.

LU$_8$ (經渠) : Ching-Ch'ū, Meridian gutter

This point is situated between LU$_7$ and LU$_9$, at 1/3 near LU$_7$.

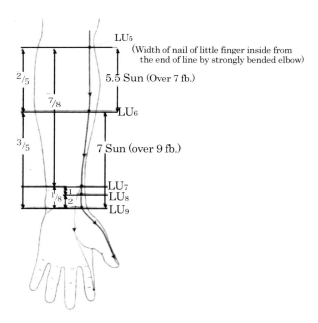

Fig.24   Points of LUNG Meridian

Attention: When seeking the points, the position of the arm should be at cardinal position, namely with stretched elbow joint and the palm upwards. By pronation, the position of points changes so much. (Fig.25)

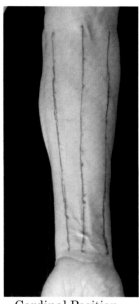
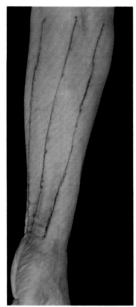

Cardinal Position　　　　　　　　　　Pronated Position

Fig.25　Deviation of Points of IN$^{(Jp.)}$(YIN$^{(Ch.)}$) Meridians by Pronation

2. Points of LARGE INTESTINE Meridian (LI)

LI$_3$（三間）： San-Chien, Three intervals
　This point is situated at the boundary of the head and the diaphysis of the 2nd metacarpus.

LI$_4$（合谷）： Ho-Ku, Connecting valleys
　This point is situated near the proximal end of the 2nd metacarpus.

LI$_5$（陽谿）：Yang-Hsi, Sunny stream
　This point is situated on the hand joint, between the tendon of long & short muscle of the thumb. This point is important as the standard point of B-cun.

LI$_7$（温溜）： Wen-Liu, Warm stagnant
　This point is situated on the line between LI$_5$ and LI$_{11}$, at the middle point between them.

LI$_{10}$（手三里）： San-Li, Three li
　This point is situated on the line between LI$_5$ and LI$_{11}$, 2 Sun$^{(Jp.)}$ (Cun$^{(Ch.)}$) (about 2.5 fb.) apart from LU$_{11}$.

50 PART 1 INTRODUCTION — OUTLINE OF ACUPUNCTURE —

LU₁₁ （曲池）: Ch'ū－Ch'ih., Bent pond
   This point is situated at the radial end of the line which appears when the elbow joint is strongly bent. This point is important as the standard point of B-cun

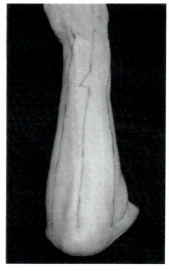

Fig.26 Points of LARGE INTESTINE Meridian

Attention: When seeking points, the position of the forearm should be at cardinal position. By pronation, the position of the points at the forearm changes markedly (Fig.27). In order to locate LI₇ and LI₁₀, it is better to mark LI₅ and LI₁₁, in the cardinal position of the arm before locating.

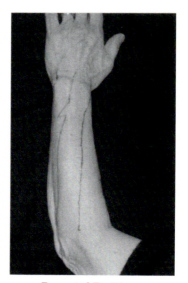

Cardinal Position   Pronated Position
Fig.27 Deviation of Points of YO-U(YANG) Meridians by Pronation

3. Points of STOMACH Meridian (ST)

ST₇ （下關） : Hsia-Kuan, Lower pass

This point is situated at the lower edge of the zygomatic process of the temporal bone, in front of the articular tubercle. This point is used for trigeminal neuralgia of NV$_{II}$.

ST₃₄ （梁丘） : Liang-Chiū, Beam mound

This point is situated on the vertical line drawn at outside of the patella, 2 Sun$^{(Jp.)}$(Cun$^{(Ch.)}$) (a little less than the width of 3 fb.) apart from the upper edge of the patella.

ST₃₆ （足三里） : Tsu-san-li, Walking three miles

There are many opinions of locating this point. Individual variation of the location of this point is often marked, and the location is not always fixed even in the same person. In many cases, this point is situated at around the point on the line between the lower end of the tibial tuberosity and the head of the fibula, about 1/3 near the tibial tuberosity. When acupoint injection hits here exactly, the patient often feels as if worms are creeping.

ST₄₃ （陷谷） : Cheh-His, Pissolving brook

This point is situated between the 2nd and 3rd metatarsus near the proximal end. It is said that the location of this point is on the line between ST₄₁ and ST₄₄, about 1/3 from ST₄₄, but the location of this point is often a little more proximal (around the center of dorsum of the foot).

ST₄₄ （内庭） : Nei-Ting, Inner court

This point is situated between the 2nd and 3rd MPJ, distal from the joints.

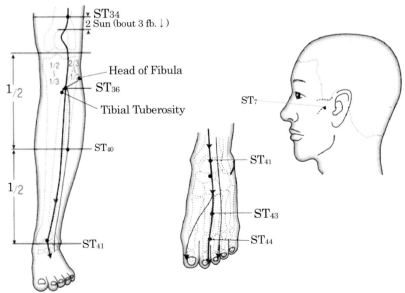

Fig.28　Points of STOMACH Meridian

4. Points of SPLEEN Meridian (SP)

SP₃ (太白) : Tai-Pai, Toowhite

There are various opinions about this point. In this book, this point is shown at under the distal end of diaphysis of the 1st metatarsus according to SAWADA's chart[3].

SP₄ (公孫) : Kung-Sun, Generation gap

There are various opinions about this point. In this book, this point is shown at under the proximal end of diaphysis of the 1st metatarsus.

SP₆ (三陰交) : San-yin-chiao, Crossroad of 3 Yin

This point is situated at the place 3 Sun$^{(Jp.)}$(Cun$^{(Ch.)}$) (about 4 fb.) apart from the medial malleolus of the tibia. This point is taken to be intersection of three IN$^{(Jp.)}$(YIN$^{(Ch.)}$)-meridians (SP, KI and LR), and the treatment of this point produces broad range of effects on the complaints.

The place of this point (although not so evident as ST₃₆) is often not fixed. Individual difference is also often observed. And sometimes bold vein lies just under the point. This point is very useful for treatment.

SP₁₀ (血海) : Hsūeh-Hai, Sea of blood

This point is situated on the vertical line of inside of patella, 2 to 2.5 Sun(Cun) (about 3 finger breadth) apart from the upper edge of patella. According to the late Dr. MANAKA, this point has same character with SP₆ and it is often called "MANAKA's San-inkou(SP₆)".

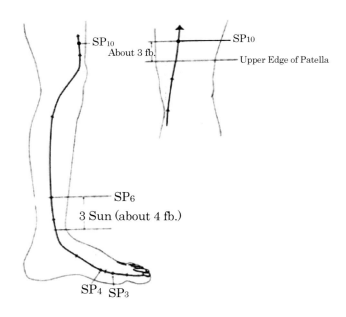

Fig.29 Points of SPLEEN Meridian

5. Points of HEART Meridian (HT)

HT₃ (少海): Shao-Hai, Young sea
　This point is situated at the ulnar end of flexor side line of the elbow joint, which appears when the elbow is strongly bent. This point is important as the standard point of B-cun.

HT₇ (神門): Shen-Men, God's door
　This point is situated at the top of the styloid process of the ulna. This place is just on the hand joint, and it is not desirable to insert needle. However, this point is important as the standard point of B-cun.

HT₄ (霊道): Ling-Tao, Ghost path
　This point is situated on the line between HT₇ and HT₃, apart from HT₇ 1.5 Sun$^{(Jp.)}$ (Cun$^{(Ch.)}$), about 2 fb.

HT₅ (通里): Tung-Li, Inner communication
　This point is situated on the line between HT₄ and HT₇, about 1/3 from HT₄.

HT₆ (陰郄): Yin-Cheh, Yin tortuosity
　This point is situated on the line between HT₄ and HT₇, about 1/3 from HT₇.

Attention: When seeking points, the position of arm should be at cardinal position, namely with stretched elbow joint and palm upwards. By pronation, the deviation of points is not negligible (Fig.25).

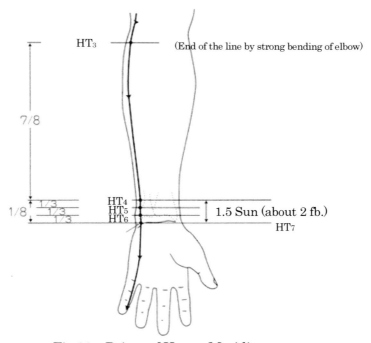

Fig.30　Points of HEART Meridian

6. Points of SMALL INTESTINE Meridian (SI)

SI₅ (陽谷) : Yang-Ku, Sunny valley

This point is situated at the top of the styloid process of the ulna, back side of the hand. This place is just on the hand joint, and it is not desirable to insert needle. However, it is important as the standard point of B-cun.

SI₈ (小海) : Hsiao-Hai, small sea

This point is situated between the olecranon of the ulna and the lateral epicondyle of the ulna. As this point is just on ulnar nerve, this point is not desirable to insert needle. However, it is important as the standard point of B-cun.

SI₃ (後谿) : Hou-Hsi, Back stream

This point is situated at the distal end of the diaphysis of the 5th metacarpal bone.

SI₄ (腕骨) : Wan-Ku, Wrist bone

This point is situated on the 5th metacarpus and carpal bones.

SI₆ (養老) : Yang-Lao, Nourishing the old

This point is situated on the styloid process of the ulna, apart from SI₅ 1 Sun(Cun) (about the width of the nail of the thumb).

SI₇ (支正) : Chih-Cheng, Supporting the upright

This point is situated on the line between SI₅ and SI₈, 5 Sun(Cun) (a little shorter than 7 fb.) from SI₅, about 2/5 from SI₈.

In order to locate SI₇, it is better to mark SI₅ and SI₈, in the cardinal position of the arm before point taking. (Fig.27).

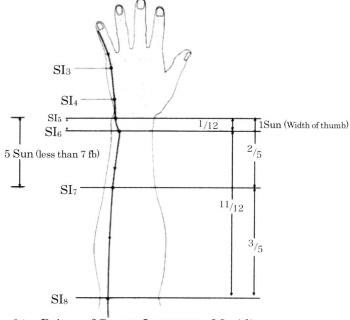

Fig.31 Points of SMALL INTESTINE Meridian

7. Points of Bladder Meridian (BL)

BL₂ （攢竹）: Tsuan-Chu, Drilling bamboo
　This point is situated at the median end of the eyebrow.

BL₄ （曲差）: Ch'ū-Ch'a, Receiving light
　This point is situated at the border of the hair, 1.5 Sun$^{(Jp.)}$(Cun$^{(Ch.)}$) (about 2 fb.) from the center line of the face.

BL₅ （五処）: Wu-Ch'u, Five locations
　This point is situated on the line which is parallel to the center line of the head through BL₄, apart about 1 Sun(Cun) (one fb. of thumb) from BL₄.

BL₆ （承光）: Ch'eng-Kuang, Receiving light
　This point is situated on the above mentioned line, about 1.5 Sun(Cun) (2 fb.) apart from BL₅.

BL₇ （通天）: T'ung-Tien, Reaching heaven
　This point is situated on the above mentioned line, about 1.5 Sun(Cun) (2 fb.) apart from BL₆.

　These points are situated at the face or the head. As mentioned before, these points are inconvenient for acupuncture. However, for the patients who have sensory paralysis of lower extremities, these points must be used. Because any kind of acupuncture therapy using points at sensory paralyzed region is ineffective.

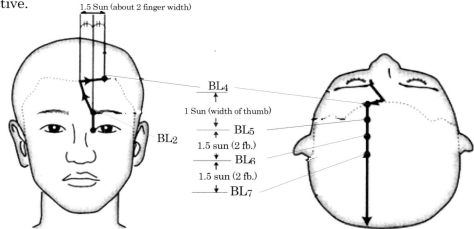

Fig 32-1　Points of BLADDER Meridian (Head)

BL₅₇ （承山）: Ch'eng-Shan, Supporting hill
　This point is situated at the junction of the venters of the gastrocnemius muscle. For the acupuncture treatment of this point, the patient must lie face down, thus it is not convenient. Thumbtack needle is mainly used here.

BL₅₈ （飛揚）: Fei-Yang, Flying expanding
　This point is situated on the vertical line which pass the posterior margin of the Achilles' tendon, almost the same height of BL₅₇

56   PART 1 INTRODUCTION – OUTLINE OF ACUPUNCTURE –

BL59 （跗陽）：Fu-Yang, Foot yang
   This point is situated on the above mentioned line, 3 Sun$^{(Jp.)}$ (Cun$^{(Ch.)}$) (4 fb.) from the lateral malleolus
BL60 （崑崙）：K'un-Lun, Kun-Lun mountains
   This point is situated around the start point of the above mentioned line. Here needle puncture is often difficult because of swelled synovial bursa.
BL64 （京骨）：Ching-Ku, Capital bone
   There are several opinions about this point. In this book, this point is shown at near the proximal end of the 5th metatarsal bone.
BL65 （束骨）：Xhu-Ku, Restrict bone
   This point is situated the distal end of diaphysis of the 5th metatarsal bone

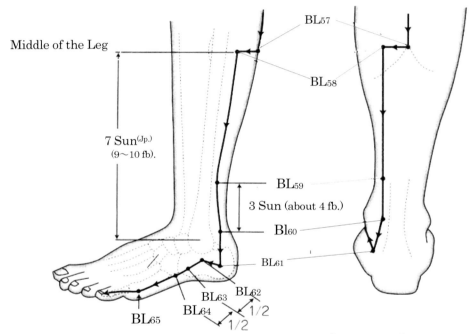

Fig.32-2   Points of BLADDER Meridian (Leg & Foot)

8. Points of KIDNEY Meridian (KI)

There are various opinions about the pathway of KIDNEY Meridian. And the location of points from KI$_2$ to KI$_7$ is often markedly different. In my practice, the following standard is used.
KI$_1$ （湧泉）：Yung-Ch'üan, Pouring spring
   This point is situated on the center line of the sole, about 2/3 from the edge of the heel. This point is not convenient for acupuncture, because patient must take face down position, the skin of this point is thick and hard, and the place of this point is not easy to keep clean.

KI₂（然谷）：Jen-Ku, Blazing valley

There are several opinions about this point. In my practice, the point at the concavity behind the navicular bone is used. In some patients, this concavity is not evident. In such cases it is difficult to detect this point exactly without search meter.

KI₃（太谿）：Tai-Hsi, Great brook

This point is situated at the back of the medial malleolus of the tibia. This point is sometimes used for acupoint injection or thumbtack needle treatment.

KI₄（大鐘）：Ta-Chung, Big ben

This point is situated at the back of the medial malleolus of the tibia, around the border of the talus and the calcaneus. This point is sometimes used for acupoint injection or thumbtack needle treatment.

KI₅（水泉）：Shuei-Ch'uan, Water spring

In my practice, the point is situated around the lateral center of the calcaneus. This point is sometimes used for acupoint injection or thumbtack needle treatment.

KI₆（照海）：Chao-Hai, Shie to sea

In my practice, the point is situated just under the medial malleolus of the tibia. This point is sometimes used for acupoint injection or thumbtack needle treatment.

KI₇（復溜）：Fu-Liy Repeating stagnant

This point is situated at the anterior edge line of the Achilles' tendon, 2 Sun$^{(Jp.)}$ (Cun$^{(Ch.)}$) (3 fb.) above the medial malleolus.

KI₁₀（陰谷）：Yin-Ku, Yin valley

This point is situated at the medial end of line which appears when the knee joint is bent 90°.

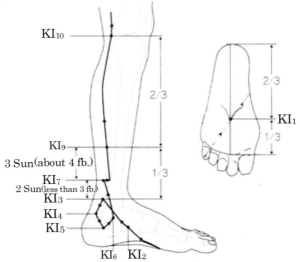

Fig.33   Points of KIDNEY Meridian

9. Points of PERICARDIUM Meridian (PC)

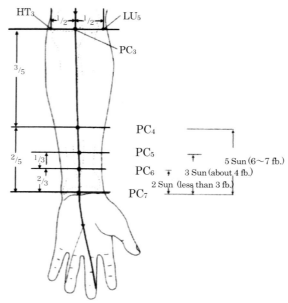

Fig.34　Points of PERICARDIUM Meridian

PC₃ (曲澤) : Ch'ū-Tze, Crooked pond
　This point is situated at the middle of the line which appears when the elbow joint is bent. This point is important as the standard point of B-cun.

PC₇ (大陵) : Ta-Lung, Great mount
　This point is situated at the middle of line at the flexion side of the hand joint. This point is important as the standard point of B-cun.

PC₄ (郄門) : Chieh-Men, Crooked gate
　This point is situated on the line between PC₃ and PC₇, apart 5 Sun(Cun) (a little more than 6 fb.) from PC₇. That is about 2/5 from PC₇.

PC₅ (間使) : Chen-Shih, The emissary
　This point is situated on the line between PC₃ and PC₇, 3 Sun(Cun) (about 4 fb.) apart from PC₇. That is about 1/4 from PC₇.
　According to the late Dr. MANAKA, this point is intersection of three IN(Jp.)(YIN(Ch.)) meridians (LU, HT and PC) like PC₆, and the treatment of this point produces effects for the complaints of broad range. This point is called MANAKA's Naikan(Jp.) (Naikan means PC₆).

PC₆ (內關) : Nei-Kuan, Inner pass
　This point is situated on the line between PC₃ and PC₇, 2 Sun(Jp.) (Cun(Ch.)) (a little less than 3 fb.) apart from PC₇, about 1/4 from PC₇. This point is taken to be intersection of three IN(Jp.)(YIN(Ch.))-meridians (LU, HT and PC), and the treatment of this point gives effect for the complaints of broad range. This point is on the tendon of superficial flexor muscle of fingers. So, careful attention must

be paid for disinfection and not to thrust tendon. In this regard, PC$_5$ is more convenient to use.

10. Points of TRIPLE ENERGIZER Meridian (TE)

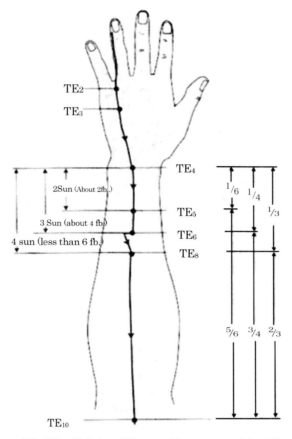

Fig.35   Points of TRIPLE ENERGIZER Meridian

TE$_4$ (陽池) : Yang-Ch'ih, Yang pond
   This point is situated at the center of the line on the back of the hand joint. This point is important as the standard point of B-cun.

TE$_{10}$ (天井) : Tien-Ching, Celestial well
   There are several expressions about the place of this point. The location of this point is on the dorsal center line, at 1 Sun(Cun) proximal from olecranon. This point is important as the standard point of B-cun. But this point is not convenient as the standard point. It may be better to seek points by the distance from TE$_4$ on the dorsal centerline of the forearm

TE$_2$ (液門) : Yeh-Men, Secration door
   This point is situated between the 4th and the 5th MPJ, distal to the joint.

TE₃（中渚）: Chung-Chū Miffle island

This point is situated between the 4th and the 5th metacarpal bone. Usually this point is regarded to be 1 Sun(Cun) from TE₂, near the border of head of the bone and the diaphysis, But often it seems to be a little more proximal. The location of this point is near the tendons. So, careful attention must be paid for disinfection

TE₅（外関）: Wai-Kuan, Outer pass

This point is situated on the line between TE₄ and TE₁₀, 2 Sun(Cun) (about 2.5 fingerbreadth, about 2/3 between TE₄ and TE₆) from TE₄. This point is taken to be intersection of three YOU$^{(Jp.)}$ (YANG$^{(Ch.)}$)-meridians (LI, SI and TE), and the treatment of this point gives effects for the complaints of broad range.

TE₆（支溝）: Chi-Kou, Branching ditch

This point is situated on the line between TE₄ and TE₁₀, 3 Sun(Cun) (4 fingerbreadth) from TE₄. This point is convenient for seeking the location of TE₅.

TE₈（三陽絡）: San-Yang-Lo, Three Yang vessels

This point is situated on the line between TE₄ and TE₁₀, 4 Sun(Cun) (about 6 fingerbreadth) from TE₄. It is said that this point is "acupuncture forbidden point". However, I have no experience of any problem by acupuncture therapy using this point. This point is also taken to be intersection of three YO-U$^{(Jp.)}$ (YANG$^{(Ch.)}$)-meridians (LI, SI and TE), and the treatment of this point gives effects for the complaints of broad range.

Attention: For point location of this meridian, forearm should be kept 90° bent cardinal position. By pronation, position of the points change markedly (cf. Fig.27).

11. Points of Gallbladder Meridian (GB)

GB₂（聴会）: Ting-Hui, Listening conference
This point is situated at the front of lower end of the tragus.

GB₂₆（帯脈）: Tai-Mai, Belt meridian
This point is situated on the anterior axillary line at the height of the navel. This point is sometimes used for the treatment of lumber pain.

GB₃₅（陽交）: Yang-Chiao, Yang crossroad
This point is situated at the lateral side of the lower leg, almost mid-point of the leg, posterior to the fibula. In some charts it is illustrated anterior to the fibula. Treatment of this point gives effect for the complaints of broad range.

GB₃₇（光明）: Kuang-Ming, Light bright
This point is situated at the lateral side of lower leg, 5 Sun(Cun) (about 6 fb. or more) from lateral malleolus of fibula, posterior to the fibula.

GB₄₀（丘墟）: hiu-Hsū、Great cemetery
This point is situated anterior to the lateral malleolus (under the anterior edge, at the height of tip of fibula). Because of synovial bursa under this point, needle must be stuck very shallow. This point is not so convenient for use.

GB₄₁（足臨泣）: Tsu-Lin-Chi, Foot coming to tears
　This point is situated between the 4th & the 5th metatarsus, near the proximal end.
GB₄₂（地五会）: Ti-Wu-Huei, Ground five meetings
　This point is situated between the 4th and the 5th MPJ, proximal to the joint.
GB₄₃（侠谿）: Hsia-Hei, Chivalrous brook
　This point is situated between the 4th and the 5th MPJ, distal to the joint

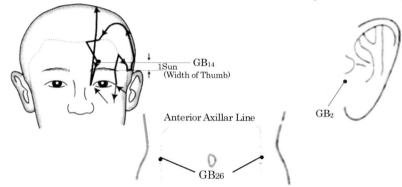

Fig.36-1　Points of GALLBLADDER Meridian (Head & Ear and Abdomen)

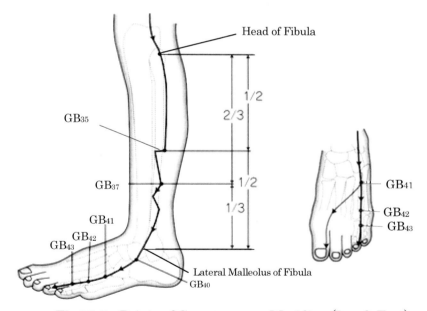

Fig.36-2　Points of GALLBLADDER Meridian (Leg & Foot)

12. Points of LIVER Meridian (LR)

LR₂（行間）: Hsing-Chien, Between colmns
　This point is situated at the medial-distal part of the 1st MPJ.

LR₃ (太衝) : Tai-Ch'ung, Great flush
This point is situated at the proximal end between the 1st and the 2nd metatarsus.
LR₅ (蠡溝) : Li-Kou, Insect gutter
This point is situated about 5 Sun(Cun) (about 6〜7 fb.) from the malleolus of tibia, posterior to the tibia.
LR₈ (曲泉) : Ch'ū- Ch'ūan, Tortuous spring
This point is situated at the medial end of the line which appears when the knee joint is strongly bent.

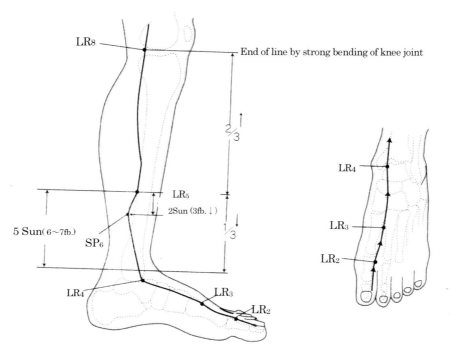

Fig.37   Points of LIVER Meridian

13. Points of GOVERNOR VESSEL (GV)

In my practice, this Meridian is seldom used except GV₁₄ and CV₂₀. For acupuncture treatment on GV₁₄, the patient must take face down position. And GB₂₀ is usually covered with hair. Both condition is very inconvenient for my method. Therefore, GOVERNOR VESSEL is used only for acupoint injection. Acupoint injection for GV14 is very useful.

GV₁₄ (大椎) : Ta-Chuei, Big vertebra
There are several opinions about the location of this point. I take this point on the spinous process of 7th cervical vertebra or between the spinal process of 7th cervical vertebra and 1st thoracic vertebra. This point is used only for acupoint injection.

GV20（百会）: Pai-Hui, Hundred meetings

This point is situated at the top of the head, on the center line of the head. Usually this part is covered with hair, so enough attention must be paid for disinfection.

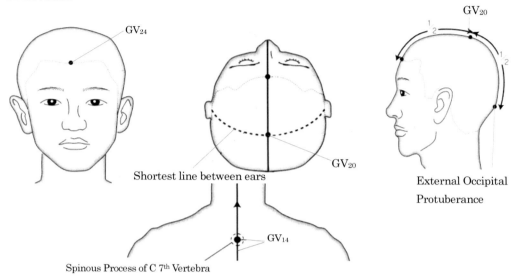

Fig.38　Points of GOVERNOR VESSEL (Back)

14. Points of CONCEPTION VESSEL

Generally points of CONCEPTION VESSEL are regarded to be important for acupuncture, and they are widely used. However, in my treatment, these points are seldom used except for the complaints of the eye (and rarely anterior region of the trunk) by acupoint injection. Most frequently used point is CV_{22}.

CV22（天突）: Tien-Tu, Sky prominence :

　This point is situated at the center of the episternum (manubrium of the sternum)

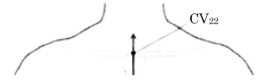

Fig.39　Points of CONCEPTION VESSEL

PART 2

MEDICAL EXAMINATION FOR ACUPUNCTURE

Chapter 1   Medical Examination of Oriental Medicine

Medical examination by Occidental Medicine is, first of all, to determine the name of the disease, and to search the cause of the disease. After confirmation of these factors, grasping the conditions of the disease, treatment is given by means of removing the cause of the disease. Medical examination is carried out along this line. Because of the marked progress of medical instruments, state of deep parts of the body, even of the molecular level, can be clarified.

The principle of the medical examination and therapy of Oriental Medicine is basically different from Occidental medicine. By Oriental Medicine, it was impossible to find out the "cause" (in the meaning of modern medicine) of the disease. And the principle of treatment of Oriental Medicine is "to check the bias of the body from the normal state" and "to let the body draw back to the normal state".

In the Oriental methods of therapy, there are pharmacologically reasonable cases such as ephedrine of ephedra herb or berberine of phellodendron bark, or methods to remove the cause of the disease in the sense of Oriental Medicine. However, here is a great difference between Occidental Medicine and Oriental Medicine. That is: the target of therapy in Oriental Medicine is not abstract "disease" but "the patient". So, the name of the disease of Occidental Medicine is almost indifferent from the method of treatment. It is not unusual to give different medicine for the patient with the same name of the disease, and vice versa.

Like the difference of therapy, the principle and methodology of diagnosis in Oriental Medicine is widely different from Occidental Medicine. The purpose of diagnosis of Oriental Medicine is not "to know the name of the disease", but "to catch the condition of the body" in order to select the methodology of treatment. Acupuncture is a method of Oriental Medicine, and diagnosis must be by Oriental method.

In the concepts of disease of Oriental Medicine, there are many factors as "stage of the disease", "IN$^{(Jp.)}$ (YIN$^{(Ch.)}$) & YO-U$^{(Jp.)}$ (YANG$^{(Ch.)}$)", "EXTERIOR & INTERIOR", "COLD & HEAT", "DEFICIENCY & EXCESS", "KI$^{(Jp.)}$ (QI$^{(Ch.)}$)/KETU$^{(Jp.)}$ (BLOOD) / SUI$^{(Jp.)}$ (WATER)", "pattern of disease according to ORGANs" etc. Combination of these factors is called "SHOU$^{(Jp.)}$ (証) (syndrome)". The plan of therapy is decided according to this "SHOU$^{(Jp.)}$". In ancient days, there were no instruments for examination, and diagnosis must be based on the practitioner's five senses.

There are four methods of diagnosis in Oriental Medicine as described below.
1 Observation
2 Hearing & Smelling
3 Questioning
4 Palpation

In the realm of Kampo[JP.] (treatment with oral medicine), the order of importance is regarded as Observation > Hearing & Smelling > Questioning > Palpation. There are not few acupuncturists who make diagnosis in the same idea. In the school of "Radical Treatment" or "Meridian Treatment", the plan of treatment is decided on the same method of diagnosis and on its interpretation same as Kampo[11][12][13]. However, this method is very difficult and it takes much time. So, in my method, diagnosis is much more simplified as mentioned later.

§ 1 Diagnosis by Observation

This is a method to make diagnosis with the sense of sight, i.e. to judge the state of patient by the inspection of figure, posture, mode of walking or color etc. of the patient. For example, according to "FIVE ELEMENT THEORY", there is a method of meridian selection according to the patient's color, as "Yellow is color of SOIL. So, yellow color of the patient indicates that the disease belongs to SOIL. THE Patient should be treated the meridian of SOIL, i.e. STOMACH Meridian or SPLEEN Meridian." But this kind of diagnosis is not so easy to learn. So, in my method, this method of diagnosis is not used. In some cases, meridian selection with Observation is possible. For example, by Herpes Zoster, meridian to be treated is evident at a glance of the location of rash.

In the treatment of Kampo medicine, judgment of deficiency-or-excess **of the body** is very important. However, in acupuncture, the meaning of deficiency and excess is quite different from Kampo. It is not so exceptional to give draining treatment of acupuncture for very weak patient. At least in my method, meridian selection by Questioning is much easier and more useful than diagnosing by Observation. The easiest and most reliable method of judgment of deficiency/excess may be pulse diagnosis. It would be better not to adhere to the appearance of Observation.

§ 2 Diagnosis by Hearing & Smelling

This is a method of diagnosis by auditory and olfactory sensation. That is, to estimate the patient's state by way of hearing the patient's voice (nature or pitch of the voice, powerful or week, condition of speaking or color of voice etc.) or smelling the patient's body odor. This factor may be useful as reference of rough information of the patient's state of deficiency or excess. But these conditions are independent of deficiency or excess **of meridian** and meridian selection.

§ 3 Diagnosis by Questioning

In Occidental Medicine as well as Oriental Medicine, questioning is very important for diagnosis. But the content of the question is widely different between the both Medicines. For example, by the treatment of cold or influenza of Oriental Medicine, in addition to common questions about symptoms, many other questions are necessary which are regarded not so important in Occidental Medicine, such as time from the onset, condition of sweating, presence of stiffness at the neck or the back, pain of the joints or the waist, time of occurrence of frequent cough, cough is dry or wet?, phlegm is heavy or weak?, expectoration of phlegm is easy or not?, presence of bitterness in the mouth, condition of fur on the tongue etc. etc., and they are all very important information for the strategy of treatment .

In acupuncture, questioning is also very important. Importance of each symptom is different according to the methodology of acupuncture. In my method, following two factors are most important.
1. What is/are the main complaint(s)?
2. Where is/are the complaint(s)?

If these two factors are vague, good effects are never obtained in my treatment.

Generally, complaints of patients are very uncertain. Not a few patients speak only what the patient convinced to be important, especially the reason of the disease or the symptoms which are not important for the therapy. In such cases, it is necessary to interrupt the patient's speech and to ferret out main complaints. When the important complaint(s) and its/their location comes to light, the acupuncture therapy can be regarded as over half successfully completed in my treatment.

§ 4 Diagnosis by Palpation

This method is also different from the palpation in Occidental Medicine. Main method of palpation in Oriental Medicine is palpation of abdomen, palpation of meridians and pulse diagnosis. In my method, pulse diagnosis is most important.

[1] Palpation of Abdomen

This method has developed especially in Japan. In the treatment with Kampo(Jp.) medicine, palpation of abdomen is very important to decide the strategy of therapy. That is to check the state of tension of abdominal muscles, resistance or tenderness at hypochondria, epigastric fluctuation, pulsation of abdominal aorta, localization of tenderness of abdomen and so on. The state of these factors are referred to decide the strategy of the therapy.

There is another type of abdominal palpation. That is to decide ORGAN to be treated from the location of abnormal findings of abdominal wall. In my acupuncture practice, these methods are not used

[2] Palpation of Meridians

This is a method to check abnormality of meridians rubbing lightly along the meridians. It may be difficult to use proficiently, and it is not used in my practice.

[3] Pulse Diagnosis

This method is very important for the judgment of deficiency or excess of the meridians. Details will be explained in the next chapter.

Chapter 2 Deficiency & Excess and Supplementation & Draining

In Oriental Medicine, deficiency/excess is very important. For acupuncture therapy, it is one of the most important factor among conditions of the disease. And it is also very important to understand that the meaning of "Deficiency and Excess" is not the same between acupuncture and Kampo[Jp.] Medicine.

"Deficiency" means "lack of something important", and "Excess" means "existence of something evil". Concept of Deficiency and Excess is not yet completely standardized. In Japanese Kampo, "Deficiency" or "Excess" is generally regarded to mean the capability of resistance against the disease (= patient's physical strength). Sometimes the word "type of deficiency" or "type of excess" is used. However, what is necessary for acupuncture is "deficiency or excess **of the meridian**".

In acupuncture "Deficiency of the meridian" means that correct KI[Jp.] (QI[Ch.]) is lack **in the meridian**, and correct KI(QI) must be supplied **into the meridian** and "Excess of the meridian" means " **the meridian** is filled with pathogen KI(QI)", and pathogen KI(QI) must be removed **from the meridian**. In Japanese, "to supply" is called "補 (ho)", and "to remove is called "瀉(sha)". There were many translated words for both words, and recently they were unified as "supplementation for supply" and "draining for remove".

It is not unusual that the state of some meridian(s) is/are deficient and the state of other meridian(s) is/are excess, and one patient is given treatment of supplementation and draining simultaneously. There is neither "type of deficiency" nor "type of excess" in the world of acupuncture.

Deficiency" and "excess" is relative estimation. Therefore, in my method, after determining the meridian to be treated, deficiency or excess of the correspondent meridian is determined usually by comparison with other meridians.

Deficiency-or-Excess of the meridian is estimated mainly by pulse diagnosis. Pulse diagnosis is also very important for Kampo[Jp.], and it is described in detail in almost all the textbooks of Kampo Medicine. There, the character of pulse is especially important. But the determination of character of pulse is extremely difficult to understand.

There are many acupuncturists who examine pulse in the same meaning of Kampo. However, at least in my method, the most important purpose of pulse diagnosis is to know "deficiency-or-excess of meridians". So, as the pulse diagnosis for acupuncture, it is almost enough if deficiency/excess of the meridians can be estimated. It is much easier than pulse diagnosis in Kampo.

Supplementation-and-Draining in acupuncture is carried out as the method shown in Table1.

Table 1 Method of Supplementation & Draining

		Supplementation	Draining
Needle		fine	bold
Method of Needle Insertion	Direction	along the flow	against the flow
	Breathing	with breathing out	with breathing in
	Speed	quickly	slowly
Stimulation	Strength	weak	strong
	Time	rather long	rather short
Manipulation		burning mountain	penetrating heaven cooling
Point		mother point	son point
Method of Needle Removing	Breathing	with breathing in	with breathing out
	Speed	slowly	quickly
	After	cover the scar	don't cover the scar
Others		(retaining needle) moxa needle (thumbtack needle)	bloodletting at well point

Chapter 3   Pulse Diagnosis

In my method of acupuncture, the purpose of pulse diagnosis is only to estimate deficiency/excess of **each** meridian. There are many kinds of pulse estimation in Kampo(JP.) Medicine, but the most convenient method for acupuncture is "Pulse Diagnosis at 6 Definite Points". This is not "only one method of estimation" even in acupuncture. There are some cases which cannot be estimated with palpation of the radial artery such as the case of amputation of the arm, A-V shunt for dialysis and so on, or palpation is extremely difficult because of the extreme abnormality of the radial artery etc., though such cases are fairly rare. Almost all cases can be dealt with "pulse diagnosis at 6 definite points".

"Pulse diagnosis at 6 definite points"[13] is a method to get information of each meridian from the pulse of radial artery. Pulse is examined on the radial artery around the styloid process of radius, with three fingers. The mode of examination is two form, slight touch and deep and a little stronger touch. From this examination twelve findings are obtained, and they are distributed to the twelve meridians. There is no such method of estimation for in GOVERNOR VESSEL and CONCEPTION VESSEL.

For the palpation, three fingers are put on the artery side by side, the middle finger on the center of the styloid process. This part is called "Middle Position (Kanjou(JP.), or Kan(JP.),)". The position of the index finger is called "Front Position (Sunkou(JP.), or Sun(JP.))", and the position of the ring finger is called "Rear Position (Shakuchuu(JP.), or Shaku(JP.),)". (Fig.40).

There are two ways of pulse examination. One method is to see pulse with very slight touch by the pad of the finger. This method is called "FU(JP.)(float)". The other method is to see pulse with a little stronger touch with the tip of the finger. This method is called "CHIN(JP.)(sink)" (Fug.41). The words "FU" and "CHIN" are used also in Kampo(JP.). But their meaning is different at all. In Kampo, these names are used as the character of the pulse, and in acupuncture, these names are the method of examination. It is very important not to mix them up. The relation between the 12 meridians and pulse at "FU" /"CHIN" & "SUN" / "KAN" / "SHAKU"(JP.), is like Table 2.

Table 2   Relation between Fu-Chin at Sun-Kan-Shaku and Meridians

LEFT			RIGHT	
FU(float)	CHIN(sink)	PART	CHIN(sink)	FU(float)
SI-Merid.	HT-Merid.	SUN (front position)	LU-Merid.	LI-Merid.
GB-Merid.	LR-Merid.	KAN (middle position)	SP-Merid.	ST-Merid.
BL-Merid.	KI-Merid.	SHAKU(rear position)	PC-Merid.	TE-Merid..

Chapter 3 Pulse Diagnosis

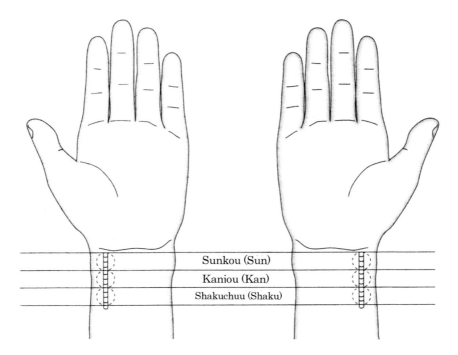

Fig.40 Position of Sun/Kan/Shaku(JP.)

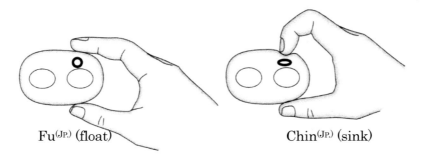

Fig.41 Manner of Pulse Taking of FU(float) and Chin(sink)

  The state of pulse change is according to the condition of the body. It changes before and after exercise, before and after acupuncture or by posture changing etc. And the estimation of the pulse is not always the same by each acupuncturist. Doctors of Occidental medicine will feel that pulse diagnosis is quite unreliable, and it is quite pardonable.

  The method to check pulse and its implication are various. The information from pulse diagnosis is not only deficiency/excess. But, here, pulse diagnosis is explained only from the standpoint of my method of acupuncture.

§ 1 Method of Pulse Taking

[1] Condition of Patient

Steady state is desirable. If possible, it is better to take rest for 10 minutes or more before the pulse examination.

[2] Posture of Patient and Position of Examiner

In my method, patient is usually treated at supine position. So, it is more convenient to examine pulse at supine position. In the treatment at sitting position such as by the thumbtack needle, pulse examination in sitting position has no problem. When the character of the pulse changes by the position, findings of pulse at supine position are adopted.

To check pulse at supine position, let the patient's hand joint put on the spinous process of the iliac bone, turning the palm upwards, and palpate the pulse in this position. The position of examiner is at the right side of the patient for the palpation of right side, and vice versa. The reason is that this position is more convenient to put fingers at right angle on the radial artery.

§ 2 Method of Pulse Examination

Right hand is used to examine the pulse of left hand, and left hand for the right pulse. Palpation is done with three fingers, index, middle and ring finger, put side by side. The middle finger is put on the middle of styloid process of radius, at right angle to the radial artery, and examine the pulse of "SUN(Jp.)," with the index finger, "KAN(Jp.)," with the middle finger and "SHAKU(Jp.)" with the ring finger. It is the same method as pulse diagnosis of Kampo(Jp.) Medicine. Then the character of pulse is evaluated: First "FU(Jp.) (float)", and next "CHIN(Jp.) (sink)".

Someone says that the pulse of both sides should be examined simultaneously, but it is not easy. It may not be always necessary to check pulse of both side simultaneously.

As mentioned before, there are vast kinds of character of pulse. In the literatures and textbooks, they are minutely explained. But it is very difficult to understand, and it may be almost impossible to master them completely by self-education. However, fortunately, the purpose of pulse diagnosis in my method is only to decide the method of treatment (supplementation or draining). So, if the character of the meridian (= deficiency or excess) is clear, it is enough useful for my method.

My method of judgment of pulse is very simple. If the pulse is weak, the meridian is deficient, and the pulse is powerful, the meridian is excess.

In the school of "Radical Treatment" or "Meridian Treatment"[11) 12) 13)], pulse diagnosis is very important for meridian selection. There, for the selection of the meridians to be treated, besides complicated diagnosis such as examination of abdomen, consideration of FIVE ELEMENT Theory etc., detailed pulse diagnosis should be taken into consideration. It is very complicated and very difficult. But, in my method, as meridian selection is decided before pulse diagnosis, judgment of pulse is only to check deficiency or excess of meridians. It is quite simple and easy.

§ 3 Judgment and Recording of Pulse

[1] Estimation of Pulse

As mentioned before, in my method of acupuncture, purpose of pulse diagnosis is only to know deficiency/excess of each meridian. And the principle of judgment is "weak pulse shows deficiency, powerful pulse shows excess". It may look too simple. But, at least these about 45 years, I have almost no experience of wrong judgment of deficiency or excess except in early days.

This method is very easy. But, for correct judgment, some training is necessary.

Pulse at "CHIN (sink)" is relatively easy to estimate.

Pulse at "CHIN" is estimated pushing artery a little strongly. Namely, it is to press the radial artery to the radius with the fingertip. If the pulse is weak, the pulsation is easily suppressed, and if the pulse is powerful, the fingertip feels repelled. It is necessary to give attention not to press artery too strongly. With too strong pressure, pulse can be estimated all deficient.

Estimation of pulse at "FU (float)" is fairly difficult. Beginners often mistake deficient pulse for excess.

The method (or knack) to evaluate pulse at "Fu (float)" is as described below.

1) To confirm pulse of radial artery same as Occidental Medicine.
2) To let finger elevate gradually not changing the position of the finger till the finger scarcely leaves skin, and examine the pulse. This state is explained "as if your finger were a fly on the artery". There is no need to mind about checking pulse of "SUN(Jp.)," "KAN(Jp.)," "Shaku(Jp.)," at once or separately.
3) If the pulse is well felt at "Fu", and the finger feels repelling by slightly stronger pressure, the pulse can be estimated as "excess". If the finger does not feel pulsation by this slightest touch, and by giving slightly stronger pressure, the finger does not feel repelling, the pulse is deficient.
4) It is necessary to take much care not to press too strongly. If the pressure is too strong, pulse can be estimated all excess.

[2] Recording of Pulse

In my method, the purpose of pulse diagnosis is to check deficiency/excess of the meridians. So, it is very important to distinguish the relation between the pulse and the meridian. It may seem very difficult. But it is not so difficult to remember contriving the form of record.

Usually the position of "SUN", "KAN" and "SHAKU" is illustrated as Fig.40. However, seeing from the examiner at medical consultation, their position is like Fig.42. "To record the pulse as it is" is the easiest method to remember the relation.

74 PART 2 MEDICAL EXAMINATION FOR ACUPUNCTURE

The design of record is like Table 3.

By the record, "deficiency" is shown with mark ↓, and "excess" with mark ↑. Writing this mark for every patient, the relation between pulse and meridian will be automatically remembered without any effort. The most important matter is to record the mark of deficiency-or-excess, not worrying about mistake. If the evaluation is obscure, it is better to give mark ↓ for the moment.

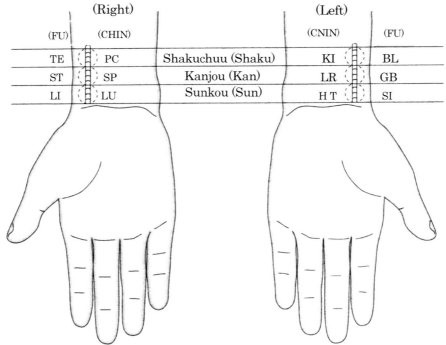

Fig.42 Six Definite Points (Sight from Operator)

Table 3 Record of Pulse

		Right		Left	
		Fu(float)	Chin(sink)	Chin(sink)	Fu(float)
Deficiency ↓	SHAKU	TE	PC	KI	BL
	KAN	ST	SP	LR	GB
Excess ↑	SUN	LI	LU	HT	SI

Chapter 4 Meridian Selection

§ 1 My Method of Meridian Selection

"To regard meridian as the most important for acupuncture" means that the first and the most important problem is "to determine the meridian to be treated".

There are many methods of meridian selection.

"Meridian Treatment = Radical Treatment" may be general consensus.

As mentioned before, by so called "Radical Treatment" or "Meridian Treatment", meridian selection is achieved after detailed Oriental medical examination.

That is: Besides detailed inquiring, after investigation of many factors such as color of the face, nature of voice, smell, diagnosis of the abdomen, diagnosis of the face and the tongue, palpation of meridians, inspection of the back, consideration on FIVE ELEMENT Theory including generating-destructive relation etc. etc., putting all these factors together, diagnostic pattern of ORGAN is decided, and then the ORGAN and meridian to be treated is decided.

This method is very complicated and difficult.

There is another method named "Ryoudouraku[JP.],". This method is to measure the electric resistance of 12 pairs of source points, and to decide the meridian to be treated on which most disproportionate point belongs. This method seems not so difficult and objectively evaluable. However, it is not so easy to detect source point, and it may take much time.

Fortunately, my entrance of acupuncture was "at first to guess the meridian to be treated, and then to treat the point of that meridian according to deficiency or excess of the meridian". There, difficult and tiresome investigation for meridian selection is not necessary. This may be one of the characteristics of my method.

It may look like "speaking without grammar". But, even by such easygoing method, excellent effects are satisfactorily obtained. In this book, only this method is explained.

The principle of my meridian selection is next four methods.
1. According to the location of complaints
2. According to the relation between ORGAN and organ &/or tissue
3. According to the resemblance between ORGAN and organ
4. According to the FIVE ELEMENT Theory

§ 2 Meridian Selection According to the Location of Complaints

This is a method to select the meridians that pass through the region where the subjective complaint exists. Headache, for example, for the pain at the occipital area BL- & GB Meridians, for the pain at the temple TE (& GB) Meridian(s), for the pain at the forehead ST Meridian etc.

This method is quite easy and useful. For this method, the most important matter is to confirm the location of the complaints. Here inquiring is the most important. As mentioned before, if the location of complaints is correctly drawn out of the patient, acupuncture therapy is estimated as half succeeded. This method is most frequently used in my practice.

After confirmation of the location of complaints, the meridians that pass through the location is sought with meridian chart or meridian doll. General charts are enough useful. But it is to be remembered that general meridian charts are not perfect. There are important meridians that are not illustrated in general charts.

Important meridians that are not illustrated in general charts are:
Brain: BL
Forehead: **ST**, TE, **GB**, LR
Temporal ~ Around the Ear: BL, TE, GB
Eye: HT, TE, GB, **LR**, **CV**
Nose: **ST**
Ear: **TE**, **KI**, **GB**, SI
Lip: **ST**, **LR**, CV
Tongue, oral cavity, pharynx: **SP**, HT, **KI**, **LR**
Around the Larynx: SP, HT, **KI**, LR
Sternal Area: HT, TE, PC
Heart: **HT**, SI, KI, **PC**
Lung: LU, LI, HT, **KI**, **PC,** LR
Epigastrium ~ Upper Abdomen: All meridians except BL & GV
Around Navel: LI, ST, SP, SI, TE, PC
Median Part of Lower Abdomen: SP, LR
Around Anus: LR, BL, KI, GV

These meridians are not always necessary. But when the effect of treatment according to the general charts is insufficient, it is worth while using these meridians together. Often marvelous effect is obtained.

§ 3 Meridian Selection according to the Relation between ORGAN and Organ &/or Tissue

In my practice, the "pattern identification of ORGANs" in the meaning of "Meridian Treatment" is not used. However, in the concept of Oriental Medicine, intimate relation is supposed between ORGAN and organ &/or tissue. Considering this relation, meridians concerning the ORGAN which has close relation to the problematic organ &/or tissue are treated. This may be curious for doctors of Occidental Medicine. But it is often very useful.

They are as described below:
1. Skin and Hair Belong to LUNG
 Apart from the problem "what is LUNG?", the fact that "swimming or rubdown with a cold wet towel is useful for the treatment of bronchial asthma" may indicate that this theory is not always absurd. Actually, for the treatment of urticaria or atopic dermatitis, treatment of points on LUNG Meridian is often very effective.
2. HEART Opens to Eye
 As mentioned before, HEART Meridian reaches the eye. For the treatment of complaints of the eye, LIVER Meridian (mainly LR$_3$) is most frequently used in my practice with excellent effect. But using points of HEART Meridian, sometimes good effect is obtained.
3. Bone Belongs to KIDNEY
 It is not credible that KIDNEY is equal to kidney. It is well known fact that kidney participates in the activation of Vitamin D. On the other hand, steroid hormones are closely related with bone. The function of KIDNEY and the adrenal body bear a striking resemblance to each other. For this theme, the latter may be more meaningful. The points of KIDNEY Meridian are used for the treatment of disease of bone such as osteoporosis.
4. KIDNEY Dominates Ear
 For the treatment of many symptoms concerning the ear, such as tinnitus, hearing loss or vertigo, treatment of points of KIDNEY Meridian is often added to the treatment of other meridians with good effect. However, this fact may be related also to the next mentioned "WATER Poisoning".
5. WATER Poisoning
 This is not the relation between ORGAN and organ &/or tissue.
 In Oriental Medicine, "WATER" means colorless liquid in the body. It likes to mean lymph fluid, but it is another concept of Oriental Medicine, and real substance of WATER is unknown.
 "WATER poisoning" is a kind of trouble of the body which is induced by excess or mal-distribution of "WATER" in the body. There are many troubles of "WATER Poisoning" such as edema, many kinds of pain, tinnitus, vertigo or bronchial asthma etc. The ORGAN that manages WATER is KIDNEY. Treatment together with points of KIDNEY Meridian promotes the effect for these symptoms markedly

§ 4 Meridian Selection According to the Resemblance between ORGAN and organ in Different Name

 As mentioned before, "ORGAN (ZOUF$^{(Jp.)}$,)" of Oriental Medicine is not the synonym of "organ with the same name of Occidental Medicine". ORGAN has two phases (morphological and functional), and sometimes the same name of ORGAN and organ seems absolutely different as SPLEEN and spleen. However, some

ORGAN seems to have correspondent organ in other name of Occidental Medicine. This is only a hypothesis. But, by meridian selection using this hypothesis, excellent effects are often obtained.

They are as described below:

1. SPLEEN

SPLEEN is evidently not equal to the spleen. Functionally, SPLEEN seems to closely resemble the pancreas. In the Spanish block, SPLEEN Meridian is called "Meridiano vazo-pancreatico (Spleno-Pancreatic Meridian)". That seems quite reasonable.

2. BLADDER

The organ that produces urine is the kidney. So, the idea that "BLADDER means the kidney?" may be feasible. Points of BLADDER Meridian is sometimes used for the attack of urinary calculus, and it is often very effective.

3. KIDNEY

KIDNEY is evidently not the kidney. The function of KIDNEY seems to be the hormone system of hypophysis-adrenal body-gonad, especially adrenal body. So, in my method, the points of KIDNEY Meridian are always used for the disease for which steroid hormone is effective.

4. PERICARDIUM

Assuming that HEART were the heart, organ that covers the heart and has some function is only thymus. The description of classic literature on PERICARDIUM[8] reminds of thymus that it is the outer membrane of the heart and concomitant with a network. Thymus has close relation with immunity. So, in my method, the points of PERICARDIUM Meridian is always used for diseases that are related to immunity or autoimmune diseases.

§ 5   Meridian Selection according to FIVE ELEMENTS Theory

Concept of IN-YO-U(Jp.), (YIN-YANG(Ch.),) and FIVE ELEMENTS is the most basic Chinese philosophy developed in the period 500 to 600 B.C.[14]. FIVE ELEMENT Theory is a concept that everything is consists of five elements, namely WOOD, FIRE, SOIL, METAL and WATER. And everything in the universe is maintained by their generating-destructive relationship. In most of textbooks of acupuncture "FIVE ELEMENT Theory" is presented in detail as one of the most important factors of acupuncture. However, this theory seems too complicated and difficult, and sometimes its argument seems sophistry. So, FIVE ELEMENT Theory is almost not induced into my acupuncture.

One exception is the use of Shikitaihyou(Jp.) (Table of Color and Body) in which various things and phenomenon applied to the Five Elements (WOOD, FIRE, SOIL, METAL and WATER). By meridian selection, Shikitaihyou is sometimes taken into consideration regarding the items described below (Table4).

1) Wind in "FIVE EVILS"

Somon[(Jp.),2] says, "When Wind is dominant, everything moves". Namely, when the "EVIL of WIND" enters into the body, the body becomes unsteady. According to this description, points of GALLBLADDER Meridian are often used for vertigo etc.

2) Tongue in "FIVE ROOTS"

Treatment of the points of SPLEEN Meridian is often effective for the complaints of the tongue. When the treatment of SPLEEN Meridian is ineffective, points of SMALL INTESTINE Meridian is used according to this description.

3) Tendon (&/or Nerve) or Skin & Flesh in "FIVE MASTERS"

In the treatment of neuralgia, stiffness or tendo-synovitis, points of GALLBLADDER Meridian (rarely LIVER Meridian) are used independent of the location of complaints.

4) Hiccup in "FIVE STRANGENESS"

Treatment of points of STOMACH Meridian is often very effective for hiccup.

Table 4 Shikitaihyou of FIVE ELEMENT Theory

	WOOD	FIRE	SOIL	METAL	WATER
ORGAN	**GB, LR**	HT, SI PC, TE	SP, **ST**	LU, SI	KI, BL
5 Evils	**Wind**	Heat	Meal Fatigue	Cold	Moisture
5 Roots	Eye	**Tongue**	Lip	Nose	Ear
5 Masters	**Tendon** or **Nerve**	Vessel	**Flesh**	Skin	Bone
5 Strangeness	Grasp	Speak	**Hiccup**	Toss	Shivering

Chapter 5   Point Selection

§ 1   Strategy of Point Selection

In almost all the literatures and textbooks of acupuncture, efficacy of each point is described in detail as its "main effect". It may be the royal road to select points according to the efficacy of points. But it is very difficult to remember all the efficacy of numerous acupoints. Furthermore opinion of each author is not always the same. The more a beginner studies, the more he will be confused.

"First to decide the meridian to be treated, and then to select suitable and **convenient** points" is my method. It is very simple and easy, and excellent effects are obtained without considering the "efficacy of points", as far as "supplementation or draining" is correct.

From ancient time, "Pivot Points" are regarded to be paid special attention at point selection. "Pivot Point" is necessary points for the specific treatment according to the type of symptoms. They are SOURCE POINT, FIVE TRANSPORT POINTS, FIVE ELEMENT POINTS, STREAM POINTS, ALARM POINTS, ACCUMULATION POINTS, COLLATERAL POINTS, FOUR COMMAND POINTS and EIGHT CONFLUENT POINTS. They commonly exist in each meridian, and they are respected to have special importance respectively. They are also described minutely in almost all the literatures and textbooks. However, excellent effects are obtained without consideration about these factors with my method.

In my acupuncture practice, supplememtation/draining is regarded to be the most important component. And, in point selection, occasionally the character of points is taken into consideration, because the character of some points has relation to the supplementation and draining. They are SOURCE POINTS, MOTHER POINTS and SON POINTS.

MOTHER POINT and SON POINT is based on the FIVE ELEMENT Theory: that is, let each "FIVE TRANSPORT POINT" in the "PIVOT POINTS" are laid out to FIVE ELEMENTS (WOOD, FIRE, SOIL, METAL and WATER) as each has the character of each element.

According to the FIVE ELEMENT Theory, there are relation of "generating relationship" and "destructive relationship" among FIVE ELEMENTS. Namely, WOOD produces FIRE, FIRE produces SOIL, SOIL produces METAL, METAL produces WATER and WATER produces WOOD (generating), and WOOD harms SOIL, SOIL harms WATER, WATER harms FIRE, FIRE harms METAL and METAL harms WOOD (destructive). The relation of them is, what produces is MOTHER of the produced, and what is produced is SON of the producer. For example, SI meridian is meridian of FIRE. Its WOOD point is SI_3 and SOIL point is SI_8. So, MOTHER POINT of SI Meridian is SI_3 and SON POINT of SI Meridian is SI_8.

For the supplementation and draining, one principle has been come down. That is "For supplementation MOTHER POINT is used, and for draining SON POINT". SOURCE POINT can be used both supplementation and draining.

SOURCE POINTS, MOTHER POINTS and SON POINTS are shown in Table 5. There are many points which are inconvenient to use. And these points are used for point selection. However, some effort is kept in mind not to use MOTHER POINT for draining and SON POINT for supplementation, **if possible** (but not so often).

Table 5　SOURCE POINTS, MOTHER POINTS and SON POINTS of Meridians

Meridian	LU	LI	ST	SP	HT	SI	BL	KI	PC	TE	GB	LR
SOURCE P.	LU_9	LI_4	ST_{42}	SP_3	HT_7	SI_4	BL_{64}	KI_3	PC_7	TE_4	GB_{40}	LR_3
MOTHER P.	LU_9	LI_{11}	ST_{41}	SP_2	HT_9	SI_3	BL_{67}	KI_7	PC_9	TE_3	GB_{42}	LR_8
SON P.	LU_5	LI_2	ST_{45}	SP_5	HT_7	SI_8	BL_{65}	KI_1	PC_7	TE_{10}	GB_{38}	LR_2

My principle of point selection is as follows.
1) "Character of points" is not regarded to be most important.
2) Convenient points for treatment are given priority.
3) Mainly points at peripheral parts of the extremities (distal from the elbow and the knee) are selected.
4) Principally points are selected symmetrically.

§ 2　Points at Auricle

French doctor Paul NOGIER expressed in 1957 on the significance of the points at auricle for the treatment. That is: In the auricle, there are many points that are correspondent to every part of the body, and therapeutic effects are obtained by stimulating these points. In China, this therapy was carried out actively since the period of the Cultural Large-scale Revolution. Also in Japan, many textbooks[15) 16) 17)] were published, but recently auricular acupuncture seems to be declining. The description of these books is not always the same, but according to any chart, good effects are expected. It is enough useful to use auricular acupuncture together with body acupuncture. Cartilage is very weak for the infection. So, strict disinfection should be kept in auricular acupuncture. This method will be explained later.

§ 3　HIRATA's Twelve Reaction Zone[18)]

This principle is advocated by HIRATA Kurakichi (acupuncturist and psychologist). That is to divide parts of the body (head, face, neck, trunk and extremities) into twelve zones, and each zone shows sensitivity of corresponding organ, and useful for the treatment (Fig.43). It seems more effective to use points that are in the zone correspondent to the aimed organ. But it is not so frequently used in my practice.

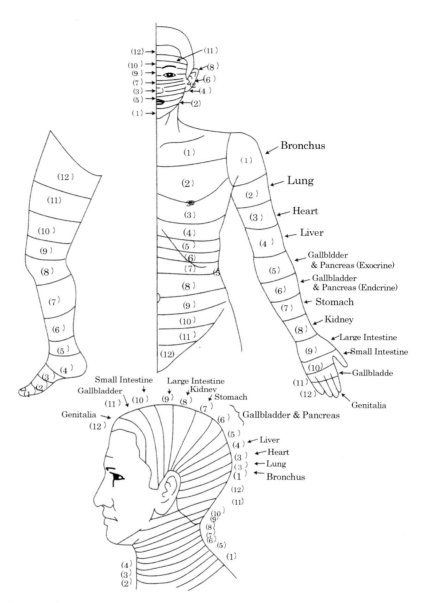

Fig.43 HIRATA's Twelve Reaction Zone[18]
(According to MANAKA's "Clinical Guide of Acupuncture"[18])

Chapter 6   Methods of Point Search

For the excellent effect, "exact hitting of needle at the points" as well as "the selection of suitable points" is indispensable. For the exact hitting, the location of exact points must be located.

In the point search, one must be pay attention that the location of points of each person is not always the same, and their expanse is also different individually. In some extreme case, the patient feels "Getting KI(Jp.), (QI(Ch.),)" at everywhere in the range of 2 to 3 cm in diameter and excellent effect appears, and in some case, the location of point is limited in the range of less than 2.5mm in diameter.

Points are located by following four methods.
1. Bone Proportional Cun(Ch.) (B-cun)
2. Electric Resistance of the Skin
3. Palpation &/or Inspection
4. Tenderness for Pressure or Puncture Pain

§ 1   Bone Proportional CUN (B-cun) (Shakudohou(Jp.))

This is a method to locate point by the distance from the standard point. Points in general meridian charts are described according to this standard. So, this method can be named "Location by Meridian Chart". This method is called "Shakudohou(Jp.)" in Japan (PART 1 § 4, p.46).

This method is the standard to determine the position of points. But the location of points is not only different individually but also it is not always constant in the same person. Acupuncture point may be rather functional one than morphological one, and it is quite natural that the location of points is often different between many literatures. I have an impression that the position of meridian chart should be treated as rough standard.

§ 2   Point Search by Electric Resistance of the Skin

Dr. NAKATANI Yoshio found that points with low electric resistance correspond with the acupuncture points in classic literatures, and the line connecting these points is closely resembles the meridian of classic literatures. He named this line "Ryoudouraku(Jp.) (Well-Pass Route)", and measuring electric resistance of SOURCE POINT of each meridian, he found that the meridian that has extremely different value of resistance is the meridian to be treated. And then he developed a method of treatment to make balance of the imbalance between meridians giving electric stimulation to the SOURCE Point of the unbalanced meridian[13]. This method is called "Ryoudouraku Therapy", which is very useful method for point location. Some instruments (search meter) are put in the market (Fig.44).

84 PART 2 MEDICAL EXAMINATION FOR ACUPUNCTURE

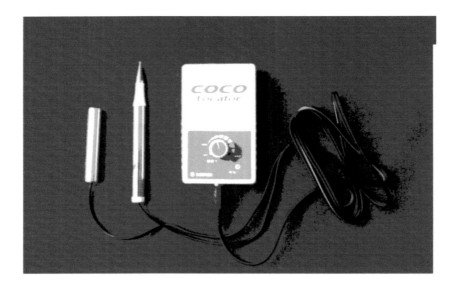

Fig.44 Search Meter ("Coco Locator")

Point location with electric resistance is a good method for beginners. However, this method is unexpectedly troublesome, and point location with this method takes much time. It is useful for beginners, but it may be a little unsympathetic for beginners. (There is a method to facilitate the use of search meter. It is to wipe around the point with squeezed alcohol swab, and to locate the point in half dry state.)

For the skilled practitioners, this method is useful for confirmation of points, especially for auricular acupuncture.

§ 3 Point Search by Palpation or Inspection

The aspect of acupuncture point has some different appearance from the surroundings. Such as small concavity, swelling, feeling of edema, too smooth or too rough, pigmentation or depigmentation etc. are often appear at the part of acupuncture point. The method of point location by this method is to touch the skin around the point of meridian chart very slightly, slipping finger, and to seek the part which has some different sensation, and to regard this point as acupuncture point. If the decision is correct, at the needle insertion "Tokki[Jp] (Getting KI (QI))" (described later) appears.

Sometimes several points with different feeling appear, and real point is uncertain. In such occasion, there is no other way to try puncture until the "Getting KI(QI)" appears. The feeling of acupuncture point will be mastered gradually in accordance with experiences.

When a point is wiped with alcohol, often the point gleams at oblique sight. Blotch, mole or decolorized spot etc. often appears corresponding with point. These phenomena are also good tool of point search. However, someone says that skin cancer appeared after injury at mole. So, points at mole would be better to avoid needling.

§ 4 Point Search by Tenderness for Pressure or Puncture Pain

Sensitiveness with pressure or puncture is one of the differences of points from the surrounding skin. When the location of point is not clear with other methods, it is good information of point location.

Next three cases are good indication of this method for point location.

1) Auricular acupuncture

Points of the ear are very difficult to detect by palpation or inspection. On the other hand, the point detected by electric resistance and the point detected by pressure pain is widely correspond each other. Pressure pain with toothpick or handle of acupuncture needle is enough useful for point location. By auricular acupuncture, puncture pain is also useful for point location. That is, to regard the painful part by slight puncture as acupuncture point.

2) Acupoint Injection

One of the merits of acupoint injection is that "good effects are obtained as if the needle does not hit the point exactly". But the effect is better by exact hitting. When the practitioner is not accustomed to point location, this pressure pain method is useful.

3) SSP [6]

As acupuncture without needle, SSP is a good method. One of its demerits is the difficulty to hit the point exactly. By SSP therapy, point search by pressure pain with the tip of SSP is very useful.

PART 3

MANAGEMENT OF NEEDLE
AND
STIMULATION & SUPPLEMENTATION-DRAINING

Chapter 1   Management of Needle

§ 1   Position and Posture by Acupuncture

[1] Position of the Patient

Theoretically acupuncture can be performed in any position, i.e. sitting-, spine- or prone position. In my practice, points on the back are not used except with acupoint injection, and spine position is mostly used. Sitting position is used only by intradermal needle or thumbtack needle treatment and acupoint injection.

Some say that spine position of the patient affects tonus of the autonomic nervous system. But according to my experiences of treatment for bronchial asthma, treatment in spine position gives always excellent effects. So, in acupuncture, the state of autonomic nervous system seems not to be affected by the position of patient so much.

Some patients cannot take supine position. If the reason is pain, he/she can easily take supine position after the treatment of acupoint injection. For the patient who cannot take spine position at any cost, treatment with electro-acupuncture or moxa needle is difficult. They must be treated with other method such as acupoint injection or intradermal acupuncture or thumbtack needle.

[2] Position of the Leg

Acupuncture on the legs &/or feet can be performed also by spine position. However, this position is sometimes inconvenient for the simultaneous treatment on the arms &/or hands. The best position for the treatment of the legs &/or feet is spine position with knee-flexion using soft pillow (Fig.45).

In this position, sometimes legs of the patient show extreme external rotation and the treatment of BLADDER Meridian becomes difficult. For this case, supporter made of elastic bandage is very useful (Fig.46). This supporter must be made of soft material.

In extreme equinus foot, treatment of BL_{60} is difficult. If correction is difficult, it is better to select other points.

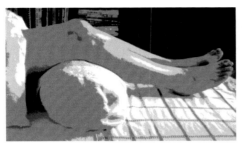 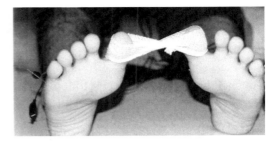

Fig.45　Position of Leg by Acupuncture　　Fig.46　Prevention of External Rotation

[3] Position of the Arm

For the treatment of the arm, the position must be placed convenient for needling and also the position must be kept during the treatment. If the treatment is limited only for IN$^{(Jp.)}$ (YIN$^{(Ch.)}$) meridians, extended (palm up) position is adequate. After needling, the patient's arm often pronates slightly, but it is almost harmless. If the patient cannot keep extended position, soft pillow under the hand joint (Fig.47) is useful.

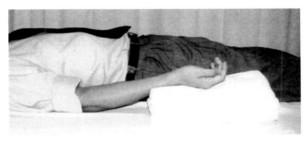

Fig.47　Prevention of Extreme Ppronation of Arm

For the treatment of both IN$^{(Jp)}$(YIN$^{(Ch)}$) and YO-U$^{(Jp)}$(YANG$^{(Ch)}$) meridians simultaneously (this treatment is fairly difficult), recommended position of the arm is "styloid process of ulna on the iliac spine". Sometimes marking is necessary (mentioned later). If this position is difficult for the patient, soft pillow under the elbow joint is useful (Fig.48).

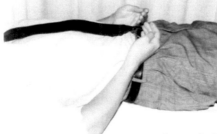

Fig.48　Position of Arm by Treatment of YO-U(YANG)-&-IN(YIN) Meridians

But, usually, in these positions, forearm of the patient is kept in somewhat pronated position. In the pronated forearm, meridians shift to ulnar side. It is not negligible. To locate correct points, the best way is to put guiding mark of meridian in cardinal position (Fig.49).

As the standard point, the following points are useful.

Large Intestine Meridian (LI): LI$_6$ & LI$_{11}$ or LI$_7$

Triple Energizer Meridian (TE): TE$_4$ & TE$_6$ (Fig.49)

Small Intestine Meridian (SI): SI$_5$ or SI$_6$ & SI$_8$

FOR SMALL INTESTINE Meridian, marking is usually not necessary except for SI$_7$. Marking is made in cardinal position of the arm. Namely, from extended forearm in palm up position, then to bend elbow 90⁰ as it is (Fig.49), and marking is made at that position.

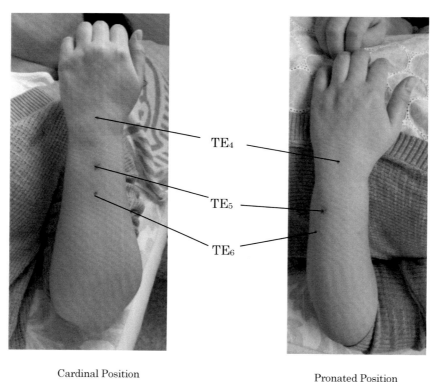

Cardinal Position   Pronated Position

Fig.49 Guiding Mark of TRIPLE ENERGIZER Meridian

[4] Position of Practitioner

For the needling of the arm or the hand, operator had better stand or sit down at the side of puncture. For the leg or the foot, the best position is between the legs of the patient. Sitting position (on the movable chair, if possible) is recommended.

§ 2 Management of Filiform Needle

Needling is usually performed as following process. Needless to say that it is very important to wash hands and to keep hands as clean as possible before needling.
① Massage of the needle insertion site (Preliminary Massage).
② Disinfection of the needle insertion site.
③ Putting the needle at the point and stick the needle into the skin (Skin Cutting).
④ Insert the needle to the necessary depth (Insertion).

The method of needle insertion is different in Japan and in China. Even in Japan, the method is not unified, and from my viewpoint as a surgeon, there are some problems on the disinfection or aseptic technique.

There are good textbooks for the practical skill of acupuncture [19][20]. But, in this book, only my method is described.

[1] Preliminary Massage

This is to seek point with fingertip (usually index finger) and to massage the surroundings of the point. With this handling, needling pain can be minimized. This technique is also useful in usual injection.

[2] Disinfection

Skin around the point should be disinfected about 3 to 4 cm in diameter. This is to prevent needle tip from contamination, as if the tip touched the neighboring skin. Some patients have very dirty skin. For such cases, "cleaning the skin before disinfection" is very important.

70% ethyl alcohol is practically enough useful as for usual injection. Management of disinfectant is same as usual injection. One swab should be used at most for two parts. Disinfected parts must not be touched with practitioner's finger.

Most part of the skin of the auricle adheres to cartilage. Cartilage is susceptible to infection. So, disinfection and aseptic technique must be performed with extreme care. In auricular acupuncture, disinfection should be strict as surgical operation. Usually, after careful cleaning with alcohol swab, disinfection with povidone-iodine is given without bleaching with hypo-ethanol.

Joint and/or tendon sheath or synovial bursa is also susceptible to infection. In such places, also strict attention is necessary.

[3] Skin Cutting and Needle Insertion

A. Needle Tube Method (Fig.51)

Horny layer of the skin is most resistant against needle penetration. To overcome this barrier, SUGIYAMA Waichi, a Japanese acupuncturist in the Edo period, invented needle tube method. This method is to insert needle through fine guide tube, so as to let the needle easily pass the strong horny layer. This guide tube is called "Needle Tube".

Originally modern needle tube is made of metal, and its management is not so easy. Recently, however, disposable needle attached to sterilized plastic needle tube is widely used. From the viewpoint of aseptic technique, disposable needle of this type is evidently better than conventional metal tube. So, in this book, only the method with this type of disposable needle is explained.

There are two types of disposable needle with needle tube. One is the tube with visible stopper, and the other is the tube with invisible function of stopper. The latter seems more convenient, but the technique to remove the function of stopper is sometimes comparatively difficult. Occasionally the function of stopper loosens, and freely moving needle tip breaks the package. In this type of the needle, attention must be paid in the function of the stopper. If function of the stopper is not intact, the needle must be scrapped because microscopic pinhole is hardly visible.

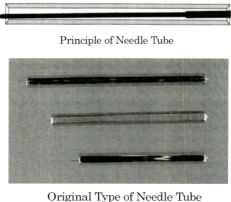

Principle of Needle Tube

Original Type of Needle Tube

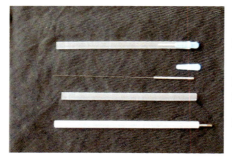

Disposable Needle with Stopper

Stopper
Needle
Plastic Needle Tube

Disposable Needle without Stopper

Disposable Needle with Sterilized Plastic Needle Tube
Fig.50 Needle Tube

The process of skin cutting is as described below.
① Hold the needle tube with the thumb and the index finger of the left hand, and fit the tip on the point. (① of Fig.51)
② Loosen the stopper or stopper-function of the needle tube with right hand. (②)
③ Fix the direction of the tube according to supplementation or draining. (③

④ Tap the top of handle of the needle with right index finger. (④)
   (This work is called "skin cutting".)
⑤ Remove the needle tube with the right hand and hold the needle body with the left thumb & index finger at the part near handle of the needle, in order not to touch the part to be inserted into the body. (⑤)
⑥ Insert needle under collaboration of the right-&-left hand. (⑥)

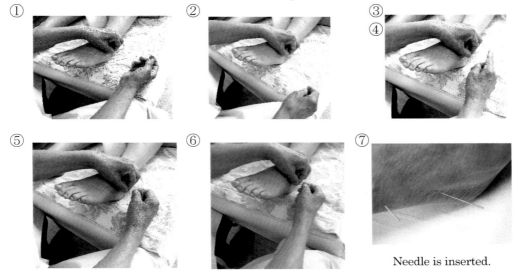

Fig.51   Skin Cutting and Needle Insertion with Needle Tube

B. Insertion without Needle Tube (Fig.53)

 · Chinese acupuncture needle has a knot at the tip of the handle. So needle tube cannot be used.
 · Using needle tube, exact hitting is difficult at extremely small point.
 · When some hindrances (such as blood vessel etc.) exist under the point, or extreme attention must be paid to avoid contamination by needling.

In such cases, application of needle tube method is difficult or impossible, and needle insertion without needle tube is necessary.

The most important point "to insert needle without needle tube" is "not to touch fingers at needle body that will be inserted into the body".

My method is as described below.

① Hold the handle of needle with the right thumb and index finger, and put the needle tip at the aimed point. ⓐ
② Pinch the needle body with the left thumb-&-index fingers. The part to pinch needle should not have possibility of entering into the body during treatment. Direction of needle is kept with the left fingers according to the purpose of supplementation or draining. ⓑ

③ Softly push the needle with the left fingers so as not to bend the needle, and simultaneously push the handle of the needle softly twisting with the right fingers, and penetrate the horned layer.

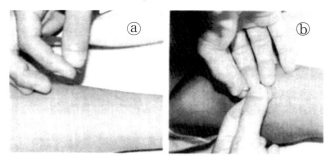

Fig.52 Skin Cutting without Needle Tube

The merit of this method is practicability of smooth transitional penetration into the skin. It seems difficult to perform, but it can be performed with some practice.

The demerit of this method is a little stronger pain than needle tube method. Usually it is tolerable. But for patients who have strong reflex, this method is often difficult to use.

Short needles less than 30mm can be easily used with this technique with the right hand only.

[4] Penetrating Needle into the Skin

This is a technique to let the needle tip arrive at the necessary depth. This technique is indispensable for acupuncture, and it is very important to acquire proficiency in this technique. Next 3 factors must be paid good attention.

1. Correct direction of the needle.
2. Finger should not touch the needle body where the needle enters the skin.
3. Send the needle tip at the proper depth.

A. Direction of the Needle

The direction of needle insertion is decided according to **Deficiency or Excess of the meridian**. For supplementation of the meridian, the direction is along the flow of the meridian, and for draining of the meridian, the direction is against the flow of the meridian. This relation is called "Geizui[Jp] (along or against the direction of the flow of the meridian)". For correct selection of this relation, it is the most important to keep needle in correct direction **at skin cutting**.

Sometimes "to keep correct direction of needle tube" is difficult because of the length of the tube. Then "Insertion without Needle Tube" must be used.

That is: after putting the needle tip at the point, the needle is given suitable curve so as to keep the needle "correct direction **at the needle tip**", and then the needle is pushed with fingers as mentioned before. Practice of this method is possible together with the practice of penetrating needle (mentioned later).

B. Prevention of Contamination

The crucial point of prevention of contamination is "Fingers should not touch the part of needle body where it can enter the body".

C. Depth of Insertion

The principle is "Till the patient feels Tokki (Good GETTING KI$^{(Jp.)}$(QI$^{(Ch.)}$) (mentioned later)". The depth of Getting KI(QI) varies point by point, and person by person. Often it is felt a few times at one needling. Very shallow puncture as thumbtack needle of 0.3mm can often cause excellent effects without Getting KI(QI). However, in electro-acupuncture, too shallow puncture is inadequate to keep needle during the treatment. So, in electro-acupuncture, usually the needle is inserted up to the depth of 2.5cm to 3cm.

D. Training of Skin Cutting and Needle Insertion

Skin cutting with needle tube is very easy. Caution in skin cutting is only to keep needle tube for correct direction. Training of skin cutting without needle is on the extension line of training of needle penetration into the skin. When the skin cutting without needle tube is easily performed, the practitioner can easily send needle into the skin every time. The finer and the longer the needle is, the more difficult skin cutting as well as needle insertion. So, it is better to begin this training using thick short needle, and to change over to training with finer and/or longer needle. As the training, following course is recommended:

First 3cm No.24, then 4cm No.24, → 4cm No.20, and then 5cm No.20. Training with 3cm No.24 can be omitted.

As the material of training, it is better to begin from soft object, and gradually promote to harder one. For the beginners, citrus fruit like grapefruit is recommended. That is to practice the training mentioned above using a fruit fixed in a suitable bowl. Next to the citrus fruit, as harder object, apple is convenient. After apple, wet gauze ball is recommended. That is to make ball of wet gauze larger than grapefruit, and to wind up the ball with strong fine thread at various strength. When "skin cutting and penetration" with 5cm No.20 (especially without needle tube) is easily possible with hardest gauze ball, this training is completed.

The knack of needle management of penetration (and insertion without needle tube) is to adjust the direction of promoting power at the needle tip to the direction of tangent line at the needle tip. Managing needle according to this principle, skin cutting and insertion with 3cm No.24 needle is easily possible with the right hand only. Usually penetration into the skin does not need twisting. When the penetration is difficult because of some resistance, soft twisting with slight pushing can help penetration. This training should be completed before actual treatment of patient.

§ 3 Getting KI(JP.)(QI(Ch.)) ("Tokki(JP.)" or "Hibiki(JP.)")

When the needle tip hits the point, peculiar sensation appears. It is a kind of unpleasant pain, like weighty, or numb or swollen or jarring on the nerve. This sensation is called "Getting KI(Q I)" or "Tokki("or "Hibiki"). When the needle tip hits point very exactly, this sensation is felt at the skin cutting, and sometimes the sensation is felt a few times during needle penetration.

This sensation often makes the patients dislike acupuncture. But the effect of patient who got this sensation is evidently better. When this sensation does not appear, it is recommended to try needle handling such as moving the needle deeper or shallower, or by twisting needle very gently. Still "Tokki" does not appear, it is better to take off the needle and to try needling again. Good point is often found around inserted point.

§ 4 Management of Intradermal Needle[7] (Fig.3, p.10)

Intradermal acupuncture is developed by Japanese acupuncturist AKABANE Koubei. This is a method of extremely shallow insertion with short needle. Usually, except in Japan, shallow acupuncture is regarded to be ineffective, and shallow needling is often used as the control of RCT. But it is complete mistake.

This is a method to stick very fine short needle almost parallel to the surface of the skin. On top of the needle, a small head is attached. There are various shape of the head. In my practice, mainly needle with flat quadrilateral head is used.

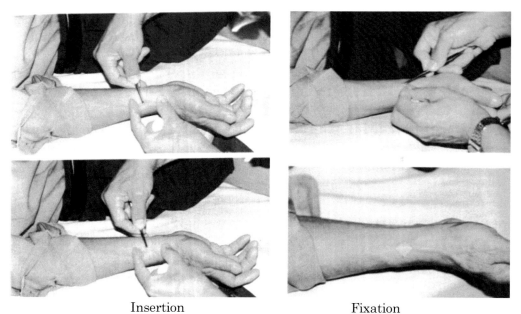

Insertion   Fixation

Fig.53   Insertion and Fixation of Intradermal Needle

Merits of this method are: .
1. Simple and convenient
2. Enough effective
3. Supplementation-or-Draining is possible

Demerits of this method are:
1. Difficult to hit point exactly
2. Fixation of needle is not easy
3. Risk of needle breakage
4. Attention for infection is more important than usual acupuncture

§ 5 Thumbtack Needle (En-pi-shin(JP.))

Thumbtack needle is also shallow acupuncture. Originally it is shaped like drawing pin (Fig.3, p11). The length of its needle is from 2mm to 5mm (or more). The greatest difference from intradermal needle is the direction of puncture. This needle is stuck vertically to the surface of the skin.

Recently separated sterilized pack is on the market (Fig.4). The minimum length of the needle of which is 0.3mm, and it is very convenient. In my practice, this Thumbtack Needle is mainly used instead of intradermal needle mentioned above.

Management of this needle itself is very easy. The order of the treatment is:
① Detect the point (if possible, using search meter) and memorize the point. (because marking is impossible except the case of using search meter, and this is the most difficult condition for the beginners), ② Disinfect the skin (photograph is omitted). ③ Open the package. ④ Take out the needle picking a part of needle mat. ⑤ Put the needle to the point and takeoff the mat. ⑥ As sterilized sticking plaster is attached to the needle, fixation is automatically performed.

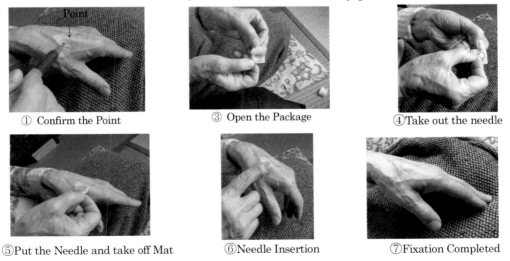

Fig.54 Application of Thumbtack Needle

Merits of this method are:
1. Simple and convenient
2. Relatively safe for infection
3. Enough effective

Demerits of this method are:
1. Difficult to hit the point exactly.

    Tokki (Getting KI$^{(Jp.)}$(QI$^{(Ch.)}$) does not appear. For the beginners, probably this method is very difficult without search-meter. Among many kinds of acupuncture therapies, difference of effects between by the expert and by the beginner may be the most evident.

2. Supplementation-or-Draining is impossible (?).
3. Intradermal needle and thumbtack needle fall out unnoticeably. In the surroundings of existing infants, risk of erroneous swallowing is not negligible.

    With this method, the longer the needle the more the risk of infection increases. Effect of longer needle may be better especially for the beginners, but use of the needle over 0.6mm is not recommended.

Chapter 2   Stimulation and Supplementation-&-Draining

There are three important conditions to get good effects with my method. They are:
1) To select suitable meridians and suitable acupuncture points
2) Correct and accurate hitting to the points
3) Never to mistake supplementation and draining

"Supplementation or Draining" is very important. It cannot be neglected. If it is mistaken, treatment is not only ineffective but reverse effects often appear. In medical conferences, there are often presentations of RCT in which supplementation and draining is neglected. Results of such kind of studies are not reliable at all.

About methods of supplementation and draining, it was mentioned before (PART2 Table 1, p.69), and MOTHER POINTS and SON POINTS (P.80) were also mentioned.

Among these factors, management of the needle and methods of stimulation is regarded as most important in my method.

§ 1   Management of Needle for Supplementation and Draining

[1] Type of Needle and Supplementation and Draining

Principle is "Fine needle for supplementation and thick needle for draining." In my practice, No.20 (0.2mm in diameter) needle is used for supplementation and No.24 (0.24mm in diameter) needle is used for draining. Finer needles are difficult to use for beginners, and they are unsuitable for moxa needle because they sag easily by slight weight. And they are also unsuitable for electro-acupuncture because of the risk of electrolysis. According to the condition, it is not impossible to use No.20 needle for draining or No.24 needle for. Supplementation.

Difference of 0.04mm is often difficult to distinguish. Distinction of thickness by the length of the needle, (5cm needle for No. 20 and 4cm needle for No.24) is convenient.

[2] Procedure of Insertion & Removing and Supplementation and Draining
Needle Insertion and Supplementation and Draining

For supplementation: Along the flow of the meridian, with **rapid expiration**.

For draining: Against the flow of the meridian, with **slow inspiration**.

In these principles, direction of insertion is the most important. Beginners often mistakes direction of the flow especially at the upper extremity (Fig.6, p14). By the mistake of direction of insertion, often the symptom becomes worse, and after correcting direction, the symptom rapidly disappears. When I was a beginner, I have experienced this phenomenon several times, and I feel that this factor may be the most important.

Angle of insertion is according to the grade of deficiency or excess of the meridian. Namely, the grade of deficiency or excess is strong, the angle is more oblique and vice versa.

Needle Removing and Supplementation & Draining

For supplementation: With **inspiration, slowly, pressing** the puncture site.

For draining: With **expiration, quickly, not pressing** the puncture site.

Observing many practitioner's acupuncture, not so few acupuncturists neglect this principle. This principle seems not to influence the effects so much. At least it may be not important as the direction of insertion. However, considering the good effect of manipulation technique (mentioned later), it cannot be meaningless.

This method does not require much effort, and it may be better to obey the instruction of predecessors.

[3] **Stimulation and Supplementation & Draining**

Like the procedure of needle insertion, stimulation is very significant for supplementation and draining. The relation between stimulation and supplementation and draining is as described below:

Retaining Needle: Supplementation (Draining is possible)
Intradermal Needle: supplementation & Draining
ThumbtackNeedle: supplementation (& Dispersion?)
Moxa Needle: Supplementation
Manipulation: Supplementation & Draining
Bloodletting: Draining
Electro-acupuncture: Supplementation & Draining
Acupoint Injection: Supplementation & Draining

§ 2   Method of Stimulation and Supplementation & Draining

[1] **Retaining Needle Method**

A. Retaining Needle

Needle puncture itself is stimulation, and retaining needle for a while promotes the effects. Method of retaining is to leave needle at the depth of deeper "Tokki (Getting KI[Jp.](QI[Ch.]). In my practice, electric stimulation is limited only at 6 points (3 pairs). If more treatment is necessary, this method is used during electric stimulation.

This method is used mainly for supplementation. So, the direction of needle is usually along the flow of the meridian. When this method is used for draining, the direction of insertion is against the flow.

By retaining needle, when the needle hits point exactly, color of the skin around the point turns white, and after a while it changes to light pink. By treatment with retaining needle only, this phenomenon is a useful information.

B. Intradermal Needle (p.10, Fig.3)

This method is to retain short and fine needles in the skin. It may be regarded to be a kind of Retaining Needle. Original method of Mr. AKABANE[7] was used as symptomatic treatment, and direction of the needle sticking was parallel to the furrow of the skin. Originally, supplementation or draining was out of consideration.

In the beginning of my practice, this method was used for supplementation. So, the needle was inserted along the flow of the meridian (vertical to the furrow of the skin). Once I had an experience of mistake. When the needle was inserted conversely, the complaint became worse promptly, and correcting the direction, the complaint disappeared immediately. This accident taught me that this method can be used both for supplementation and draining, and the importance of the direction of needle insertion. One demerit of my method of intradermal needle is a risk of needle breakage if the insertion site is movable part.

C. Thumbtack Needle (Drawing Pin Shaped Needle)s (Fig.4, p.11)

The direction of the needle is always vertical to the meridian. So it is impossible to control supplementation or draining. But actually it is effective in many cases regardless of deficiency and excess of the meridian, following the principle of my meridian-based method. Separately packed sterilized thumbtack needle (recently developed, Fig.4, p11) is very convenient to use.

[2] Moxa Needle[21]

This method is invented by Mr. SASAGAWA Tomooki and published in 1931. The method is to burn moxa on the handle of acupuncture needles. This method is very useful for supplementation. This method is concerned if it is inadequate for "Heat Syndrome". However, it is very rare case. I have no experience of embarrassment by such condition. Method of management will be mentioned later (p115)

[3] Manipulation (cf. Part1 p.6)

There are several methods of treatment with needle alone. These are collectively called "manipulation". They are as described below.

1) **Rapid insertion & removing:** After insertion remove needle rapidly.
2) **Scattering Needle:** This is to repeat "Rapid insertion & removing". The method to stick needle in several directions of definite depth is also called "scattering".
3) **Snapping Needle:** This is to flip the retained needle with finger.
4) **Twisting Needle:** This is to twist the handle of inserted needle.
5) **Sparrow Pecking Method:** This is to lift and thrust the inserted needle finely like a sparrow pecks food.
6) **Burning Mountain Method:** This will be mentioned later (p.100)
7) **Penetrating Heaven Cooling Method:** This will be mentioned later (p.101)

Among methods mentioned above, from 1) to 5) are generally used often.

"Burning mountain method" and "Penetrating heaven cooling method" are methods to perform supplementation & draining with manipulation. It is sometimes used in my practice. Procedure of this technique is not always same among practitioners. In my practice, the method of Dr. MANAKA[18] is used.

The procedure of these methods is as described below.

Burning Mountain Method (Fig.55):

This method is used for supplementation according to the following order.

① Respiration is carried out as to inhale from the nose at once and to exhale dividing 5 times from the mouth.
② Needle is inserted rapidly with exhalation till shallow layer (HEAVEN Layer)
③ At the part where "Tokki[Jp.]" is felt, the needle is twisted 3 to 9 times for the same direction.
④ Then the needle is moved forward to the middle layer (HUMAN Layer), and at the part where "Tokki" is felt, the needle is twisted 3 to 9 times as before.
⑤ Then the needle is moved to the deep layer (EARTH Layer), and the needle is twisted 3 to 9 times as before.
⑥ Then the needle is pulled back to the HEAVEN Layer, and the needle is removed slowly, and immediately the pierced part is pressed with finger.

By successful treatment, the patient feels warm sensation around the pricked part or at whole body.

In the techniques mentioned above, control of respiration may have enough meaning. However, it is difficult to let patient understand this method. Without control of respiration, almost always excellent effects are obtained

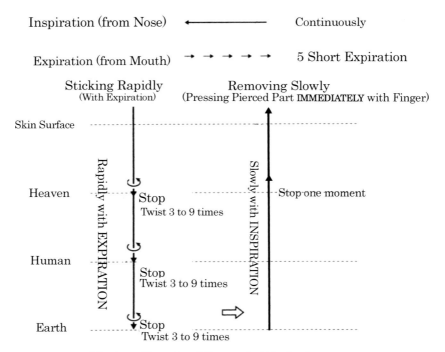

Fig.55   Burning Mountain Method
(According to MANAKA's "Clinical Guide of Acupuncture"[18])

Penetrating Heaven Cooling Method (Fig.56):
This method is used for draining according to the following order.
① Respiration is carried out as to inhale from the mouth at once and to exhale dividing 5 times from the nose.
② Needle is inserted with inhalation slowly till deep layer (EARTH Layer)
③ At the part where "Tokki" is felt, the needle is twisted 6 times for the same direction.
④ Then the needle is pulled back till the middle layer (HUMAN Layer) rapidly and inserted slowly repeating 3 times.
⑤ Then the needle is pulled back to the shallow layer (HEAVEN Layer), and the needle is left stay there for a while.
⑥ The needle is pulled out rapidly with exhalation, without pressing the inserted part.

By the successful treatment, the patient feels cool sensation around the insertion part or at whole body.

Without respiration control, almost always excellent effects are obtained.

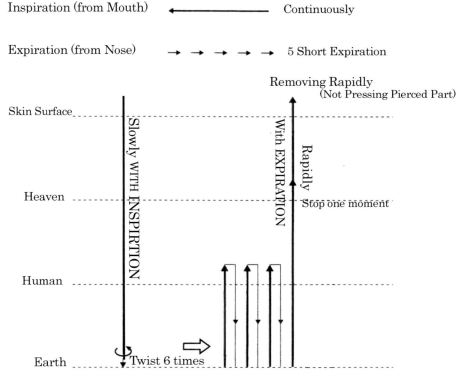

Fig.56 Penetrating Heaven Cooling Method
(According to "MANAKA's Clinical Guide of Acupuncture"[10])

The most evident demerit of these methods is pain, especially by needle twisting.

[4] Bloodletting

Treatments with bleeding are called "Blood Letting". Usual method of "Blood Letting" of acupuncture is to make bleeding by puncture of vein at head, neck, back, popliteal fossa, fingertip etc. with a thick needle. A method to let leech suck blood is included in this method. Sometimes cupping glass is used. There is a special needle for bloodletting named three-edged needle, but thick injection needle is enough applicable.

In my practice only puncture at the tip of fingers (WELL POINT) is used.

Bloodletting at WELL POINT

WELL POINT is a place where $KI^{(Jp.)}$($QI^{(Ch.)}$) of meridian arises. It is compared to the spring, the beginning of the river. They are located at the tip of fingers and toes, and they are regarded to be the place where meridians take contact with the outside world. Bloodletting at WELL POINT is to stick these points and to make bleeding.

The method is very simple. It is only to stick the WELL POINT with suitable needle, and to leave bleeding. Effects appear immediately. However, as patients with excess of meridian are relatively few, the chance to practice this method is not so frequent. Pain by puncture is a demerit of this method.

[5] Electro-acupuncture

This is a method to give electric stimulation. It is also called "Electric Acupuncture" or "Electric Meridian Therapy". Usually spike wave or rectangular wave is used for stimulation. As the frequency of stimulation, regular frequency, compressional wave or 1/f fluctuation is used. By most of instruments, stimulation is applied between two needles. From the viewpoint of stimulation control, this type is very inconvenient. Static electricity can be used as stimulation too, but usually method of this type is not included in electro-acupuncture.

Electro-acupuncture is much more convenient than manipulation in the following conditions.

1) Handling is easy and not troublesome.
2) This method can be continued for long time.
3) Strength of stimulation can be easily controlled.
4) Quantitative comparison is possible to a certain extent.
5) Less painful.
6) Simultaneous stimulation for many points is possible and it is useful for time-saving.

This method can be used both for supplementation and draining. Detailed explanation will be mentioned later in Part 4 (p.109).

Electro-acupuncture is my basic method. All the methods of acupuncture in this book are application of my electro-acupuncture.

[6] Acupoint Injection[22]

This is a method to inject some substances to acupuncture point (acupoint). This method is also called "Meridian Point Injection", "Point Injection", "Water acupuncture" or "Pharmaco-acupuncure". This method is widely carried out in many countries. But in most of them, important problem seems to be the substance to be used as vitamins, extract of placenta or bee venom and so on, and points to be used seem out of discussion.

Acupuncture is a kind of therapy to give some stimulation to inserted needle at suitable acupuncture points (acupoints). My method is similar to my electro-acupuncture, changing acupuncture needle to injection needle and electric stimulation to stimulation of injection. So, the method of meridian selection and point selection is quite the same as my electro-acupuncture, and the injected substance is out of consideration in most cases.

This method has many merits as follows.

1) **Simple and easy**. Necessary instruments are injection syringe of 1ml or 2ml and fine injection needle. In most cases substances for injection are out of problem. Any substance can be used so far as it can be used subcutaneously or intramuscularly.
2) **Excellent effects**. If the injected substance has pharmacological effect for the disease or symptom, the pharmacological effect appears more rapidly and stronger with less dose, and the effect continues much longer.
3) This method can be used even **without consideration of supplementation or draining** with good effects.
4) Good effects are obtained as if the needle does not hit points exactly.
5) **Everybody** who has authority to make injection **can easily use** this method.
6) This method may be **good entrance** to acupuncture.

Only one demerit is pain by injection. Sometimes it becomes great barrier.
Detailed technique will be explained later in PART 4 (p.121).

§ 3　Frequency of Acupuncture Therapy and Attention after Treatment

[1] Frequency of Acupuncture Therapy

It is not exceptional that the complaints disappear at the first treatment. In such case, further treatment is not necessary. In other cases, only very few patient needs daily treatment. In the major cases, treatment is necessary "when the patient feels necessity of treatment".

When regular treatment is necessary, the effect differs according to the frequency of treatment. Mostly, the difference is remarkable between less than once a week to once a week, and once a week to twice a week. Difference between twice a week and thrice a week is often not remarkable.

[2] Attention after Acupuncture Treatment

After the auricular acupuncture, especially after retaining thumbtack needle, attention for infection is extremely important. In other kind of acupuncture, there is no need to add any disposal after alcohol disinfection. Neither bleeding nor bruise after subcutaneous bleeding has to be worried. Bleeding can be stopped with pressure for several minutes, and bruise surely disappears after a few weeks. It is better to explain this accident well, because some patients worry themselves about bruise.

After acupuncture therapy, many patients feel comfortable and languid like after the bathing. Usually patients are recommended not to take a bath and alcoholic drinks at the night after acupuncture. After acupuncture therapy, many patients feel comfortable being relieved from complaints, and carelessly work too hard the next day, and feel heavy fatigue. So patients are also recommended not to work too heavy the next day. (With acupoint injection, intradermal acupuncture and thumbtack needle, this caution is not necessary.)

Once I treated a patient of facial spasm with excellent effect. Later he received electric massage at a barbershop, and the facial spasm recurred immediately. It was easily cured with the same acupuncture treatment. I thought that this patient may have received reverse treatment of supplementation-or-draining by electric massage. Thereafter I used to recommend patients not to receive electric massage or low frequency electric treatment after acupuncture therapy.

PART 4
MY METHOD OF ACUPUNCTURE

The fundamental principle of my acupuncture is electro-acupuncture with filiform needle by the following method.
1) Treating points are on the meridians that pass the area of complaints. (There are some exceptions)
2) Points are selected distant from the area of complaints, principally at the extremities distal from the elbow and knee joint.
3) Points are selected bilaterally.
4) Basic method is electric stimulation of rectangular wave.
5) Supplementation or draining is performed according to Deficiency or Excess **of the meridian,** taking balance of the stimulation.

For the electric stimulation, the instrument "Tokki" (made in Japan) is used.

This instrument has 6 channels and the strength of stimulation can be controlled by each channel. So it can stimulate 3pairs of points electrically taking balance. If the treatment is necessary more than 3 pairs, those points are treated by retaining needle, moxa needle, manipulation or acupoint injection and so on.

Auricular acupuncture is used together with body acupuncture, for diseases of joints, diseases of the eye, dental pain and so on. Auricular acupuncture is used also for the treatment of obesity independent of the body acupuncture. Eyelid acupuncture is used mainly for the treatment of motor paralysis together with body acupuncture.

Intradermal needle and Thumbtack needle are used for almost the same indications of electro-acupuncture as simple acupuncture, and also as supplemental use for body acupuncture.

Acupoint injection is used for almost all objects of acupuncture with excellent effects. Especially it is very useful for pain sedation (above all for cancer pain), bronchial asthma, pollinosis or dermal diseases. It is also useful when time is lacking for electro-acupuncture, for predicting the effect of acupuncture or as supplemental use of other acupuncture therapy.

When the needle insertion is difficult, SSP can be used, and as the most simplified acupuncture, finger pressure for acupuncture point is often used.

In this part, my method of acupuncture will be explained minutely.

Chapter 1   Medical Examination for Acupuncture

§ 1   Inspection

In the four Oriental medical examinations (inspection, auscultation & olfaction, questioning and palpation), usually inspection is regarded as most important for meridian selection. Some schools of acupuncture as "Radical Treatment" or "Meridian Treatment" attach great importance to inspection. However, in my method, inspection is used only for reference of meridian selection (by treatment of dermal diseases or fistula etc.) and to check the local symptom of heat in order to check indication of moxa needle.

§ 2   Auscultation & Olfaction

Only intensity of the voice is paid attention. When the voice is weak, the patient is given weaker and shorter stimulation as if the pulse shows excess of the meridians. When the therapy is effective, voice of the patient grows stronger.

§ 3   Questioning

Questioning is particularly important in my method. Especially next three questions are indispensable.
1) What are the patient's complaints? And what is the chief complaint(s)?
2) Ranking of the importance of complaints.
3) Location of the complaint(s).

Usually patients have a marked tendency to overemphasize what they regard to be important, and they don't tell us really important information. Some say that "In acupuncture therapy, it is very important to listen to the tales of patient, and that is one of the strong points of Oriental Medicine". However, only to listen to the patient's tale is only to take time in vain. Excellent questioning is, at least in my acupuncture therapy, not "open question" but "closed question".

In my method, "cause of disease (or symptom)" is almost needless for the treatment. And yet many patients are eager to explain the "cause" of their complaints almost of which is not "real cause". "Listen to the patient's why" is only useful for the communication with the patient.

At the questioning, the most important thing is to get the chief complaint. This is the most important factor to determine the strategy of therapy, and if the chief complaint is uncertain, my method of acupuncture is never successful. But it is unexpectedly difficult to confirm the chief complaint.

Usually questioning is performed in the following order.
① Question: What do you want to cure with acupuncture?
② Let the patient enumerate all the complaints.

③ Confirm that the patient has no other complaints.
④ Let the patient tell the most important **one** complaint.
⑤ Let the patient enumerate the order of importance of the complaints.
⑥ Ask the patient if something to be informed remains.

IN the matters that the patient wanted to inform, occasionally (not so often) some useful hint for therapy is found. So, it is better to ask this "Question ⑥".

With these questions, rough strategy of therapy is decided.

After confirmation of chief complaint, related questions are added. In these questions, "**location of the complaints**" is very important. For the confirmation of the location of complaints, it is very important to let the patient indicate the place **with the patient's one finger.** Meridian doll is convenient for this purpose. It is also important to confirm the location again finally.

§ 4   Palpation (cf. PART2 Chapter3)

As the palpation for the diagnosis for acupuncture therapy, in my method, only pulse diagnosis (p.70) is used. Diagnostic palpation of abdomen that is habitually used by the school of "Meridian Therapy" is very difficult.

In my method, purpose of pulse diagnosis is only to judge deficiency or excess of meridians. By judgment of deficiency or excess, it is also important to compare the pulse with other meridians. For the meridian of deficiency, draining is never given. However, seemingly excessive pulse is occasionally weaker than pulse of other meridians. In such rare case, sometimes supplementation is given to "seemingly excessive" meridian.

Pulse diagnosis is not used for meridian selection. In my method, pulse diagnosis is next to the meridian selection for the planning of treatment. This order of planning may be one of the most different points from other schools.

§ 5   Meridian Selection (cf. PART1 Chapter4)

The first principle of my meridian selection is "to select meridians which pass through the location of complaints". Selection of this type is most frequent. So, in such cases, when the condition of "what is the complaint to be cured?" and "where is (are) the complaint(s)" are clear, meridian to be treated becomes automatically clear. There are other principles of meridian selection as mentioned before.

When several meridians are necessary for the treatment, meridians are selected according to the importance of the complaints

§ 6 Point Selection and Point Taking (cf. PART1 Chapter5)

In auricular acupuncture and eyelid acupuncture, points are automatically determined according to the purpose of the therapy. In body acupuncture, after meridian selection, points to be treated must be selected. About point selection, it is mentioned before (p.80). Basically, "convenient points for needle insertion" on the aimed meridian is selected. It is enough useful for the treatment independent of the "character of the point". Points are selected at extremities distal from the elbow and the knee joints, avoiding points near the place of complaints. When the treatment is less effective than predicted, MOTHER- or SON points (p.80) &/or HIRATA's 12-zones (p.81) can be considered. However, for the good effects, it seems more important to select suitable meridian, to hit needles at correct points and not to mistake supplementation or draining.

Points are selected almost always bilaterally. This is very useful for the control of strength of the stimulation. "Treatment for points of opposite side" very often produces excellent effects. Bilateral point selection may be reasonable also from this viewpoint.

The number of treating points is the less the better. In my method, mainly 3 to 6 pairs of points (except intradermal needle, thumbtack needle and acupoint injection) are used. When treatment of many meridians is necessary, the "multipurpose" points as SP_6, SP_{10}, PC_5, PC_6, GB_{35} etc. are very useful.

Chapter 2 Treatment with Filiform Needle

(Body Acupuncture)

§ 1 Needle Insertion (cf. PART3 Chapter1)

Technique of needle insertion is minutely mentioned before (p.89).
The procedure is:

① Select needle of No.20 (0.20mm in diameter) or No.24 (0.24mm in diameter) according to deficiency or excess of the meridian. (It is not strictly necessary.)

② Select the direction of insertion (along or against the flow of the meridian) according to deficiency or excess of the meridian.
If deficiency or excess is not clear, it is better to insert fine needle vertically.

③ Put the needle forward until the patient feels the deepest "Tokki$^{(Jp.)}$ (Getting KI$^{(Jp.)}$ (QI$^{(Ch.)}$))".
Angle of insertion is according to the degree of deficiency or excess.
Needle for moxa needle must not be inserted too oblique.

§ 2 Electro-acupuncture (Electric Acupuncture)

[1] Principle
A. Supplementation & Draining with Electro-acupuncture
1) **Strength of Stimulation:** Principle is:
  Rather weaker for supplementation
  Rather stronger for draining.

Sensitivity for stimulation is extremely different from patient to patient. The difference of sensitivity is over 100 times! So, the strength of stimulation must be estimated by subjective sensation. If the patient feels the stimulation too strong, it is too strong stimulation as if concrete numerical value is weak, and vice versa.

"Adequate stimulation is what the patient feels comfortable" is a mark of stimulation. Often the patient sleeps during treatment, and excellent effects seems to appear more often by such patients. It is quite simple, but this standard may not be irrelevant.

2) **Time of Stimulation**

Standard stimulation time is from 15 to 25 minutes for supplementation and from 10 to 15 minutes for draining. Patients of new injury need relatively strong and very long time stimulation (sometimes over 1 hour) like acupuncture anesthesia.

3) **Frequency of Electric Stimulation**

According to the oral teaching of the late Dr. MANAKA, "Low frequency for supplementation, and high frequency for draining. The border is 60Hz". Obeying the Dr. MANAKA's instruction, the stimulation is adopted 3Hz for supplementation and over 125Hz for draining.

4) When Judgment of Deficiency-or-Excess of Meridian is Uncertain

Usually there is a tendency that "patients with deficiency cannot endure strong stimulation, and patients with excess don't feel weak stimulation". When the patient is too sensitive or too insensitive for stimulation than expected, it is worth reconsidering if the pulse diagnosis was wrong. But this is not absolutely applicable. After all, pulse diagnosis is most reliable for the judgment of deficiency or excess of the meridians.

Beginners are often confused with the judgment of deficiency or excess of the meridians. "When deficiency or excess is uncertain, treat the patient as deficiency!" is common sense of Oriental Medicine. Especially with pulse diagnosis of YO-U$^{(Jp.)}$ (YANG$^{(Ch.)}$) Meridians, beginners have tendency to mistake the character of meridian as excess. There is one method to treat patient of uncertain pulse diagnosis. That is to use fine needle (No.20) with vertical insertion, and to give the patient 45Hz stimulation. If the patient likes weak stimulation the patient is treated as deficiency, and vice versa

5) When Simultaneous Use of Supplementation & Draining is Necessary

In treatment with Kampo$^{(Jp.)}$ Medicine, formulas for supplementation and for draining are never used simultaneously. But, in acupuncture, it is common to treat some deficient meridians for supplementation and to treat other excess meridians for draining. Principle of treatment for such case is as mentioned below.

1. Treatment of the most important meridian is mentioned everything above.
2. Draining is given priority of electric stimulation.
   Supplementation treatment is given by retaining needle or moxa needle for lack of channels.
3. If simultaneous electric stimulation of supplementation & draining is necessary, it is distinguished by thickness of needles, direction of insertion and mode of insertion and removing. Stimulation is given with 45Hz rectangular wave.
4. If the meridians to be drained are over 3 pairs, left meridians are treated with retaining needle, manipulation or acupoint injection.

B. Balance of Stimulation

Balance of stimulation is regarded as important as (or more than?) strength of stimulation. That is to take balance of stimulation so as that the patient feels the strength of stimulation equal at every (at least one pair of) point.

When balance taking is extremely difficult, there is nothing but to continue imbalanced stimulation. In this case, stimulation control should be aimed at the most strongly felt point. It is to control stimulation so as the patient does not feel unbearable. During such stimulation, often the balance improves by degrees.

It may be very difficult to give adequate stimulation with manipulation without severe training under excellent leader. The "well balanced comfortable electric stimulation" may be the most simple & easy adequate stimulation.

[2] Instruments for Electric Stimulation

Many kinds of instruments for low-frequency electric stimulation are on the market. Most of them are installed channels that have two poles with wire to connect with acupuncture needle. Instruments of this type cannot control the strength of stimulation of each needle. Instruments of this type are not suitable for my method.

Electric Stimulator "Tokki" (Fig.57)

An instrument, strength of stimulation of each channel of which can be controlled separately is available in Japan. Its name is "Tokki".

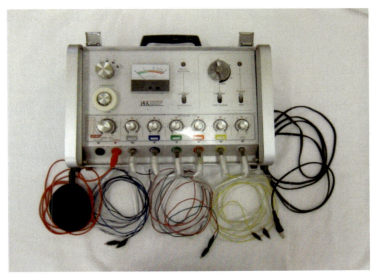

Fig.57   Electric Stimulator "Tokki" (Type Ⅲ)

A. Structure and Merits of "Tokki"

"Tokki" is an instrument to produce cathode rectangular wave. Anode plate made of conductive rubber is used as indifferent electrode. "Tokki" has main controller and six electrode channels, and each channel has variable resistor respectively. So, the strength of stimulation can be controlled totally and separately at each channel.

Five kinds of frequency, 1Hz, 3Hz, 10Hz, 45Hz and 125Hz are equipped. Power source is 100V for home use electricity.

Needle breakage due to electrolysis is the most troublesome complication of electro-acupuncture. Electrolysis appears at anode. By this instrument, needle is always stimulated at cathode, and it is free from the risk of electrolysis. This is also the merit of this instrument.

B. How to Operate "Tokki"

My method of operation is:

① to put indifferent electrode plate on the body previous to needle puncture,
② after needle insertion, electric cord is connected with each needle,
③ adequate electric stimulation is given
④ regulating strength at each needle during adequate time.

The procedure is as described below.

1) Put Indifferent Electrode Plate on the Body

There are many opinions about the position of indifferent plate. Actually, it seems that the place of the indifferent electrode gives no influence for the effect. By the spine position, "at back" (under the body) seems most convenient. Plate must be put before needle insertion, and it must be attached directly on the skin.

2) Connect Electric Cord with Needle

Light electric cord and clip, as light as possible, is desirable.

It is recommended to make pairs and to divide pairs with plastic tube etc. (Fig.57). It is convenient not only for keeping cords but also for the control of stimulation. Each cord has different color. It is recommended to form the habit to use fixed colors for right or left side of the patient.

It is better to connect clip with handle of needle. Needle with plastic handle or glued handle, clip has to be connected with needle body. But it is not desirable because of instability of fixation and insecurity of disinfection. Considering the use of moxa needle, needle with welded or pressure bonded handle is necessary.

Occasionally needle drops out because of the weight of electric cord or clip. This "drop out" can be prevented by fixing cord and the skin with sticking plaster. In auricular acupuncture or eyelid acupuncture, this method is indispensable.

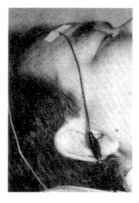

Fig.58   Fixation of Electric Cord with Skin

3) Stimulation

Stimulation given to patients needs to be with adequate frequency and strength, during suitable time as mentioned before. Standard strength of my method is as "the patient feels comfortable", and for supplementation rather weak and for draining rather strong, but never let patient feel pain.

4) Control of Strength of Stimulation

Ideal control is that the patient feels the stimulation of each channel equal. "Tokki" has 6 channels that can be controlled separately. But it is often difficult to keep balance of stimulation of each channel. My usual procedure is as described below:

① Let the switch of every channel set minimum.
② It is very important let the patient never to move extremities, and answer the question only orally. Question must be very simple. The best question is to be able to answer with yes-or-no.
③ Intensify the main switch slowly, and tell the patient that when some stimulation is felt say "I feel!". At that time, never tell the patient "where did you feel?" This question is likely to cause movement of the arm &/or hand.
④ When the patient begins to feel stimulation, the location of most strongly felt stimulation is confirmed, and the strength of stimulation at the pair is regulated to be balanced. Question must be very simple as to be answered with one word, as "arm or leg or foot?", "right or left?", "too strong?" etc. so as to be answered with one word. At that time, it is also important not to ask patient "where?" as mentioned before.
⑤ After taking balance of the most strongly felt point, stimulation of one of the remaining two pairs is regulated as before.
⑥ The remaining one pair is regulated as before.
⑦ Finally strength of stimulation is regulated so as to be felt equally and comfortably, hearing "isn't the stimulation too strong?", "is somewhere especially strong?", "is somewhere especially weak?"

Thus the control of stimulation is completed.

5) Art of Regulation of Stimulation

Control of stimulation mentioned above is not always easily performed. But following "arts" will help to make regulation easier.

1. Fundamental principle is to balance one pair. As if total balance is difficult, good effects are obtained so long as each pair is well balanced.
2. Basic principle of regulating balance is to reduce the stimulation of stronger channel. A phenomenon is often observed that by strengthening one channel, the patient feels as if stimulation of opposite channel is weakened and vice versa. Namely, to weaken stimulation of one channel is equal to strengthen the

stimulation of opposite pair channel. It is much better to control stimulation by weakening the stronger channel as far as the room of weakening remains.
3. One of 6 channels must be always kept minimum scale.
4. When the regulation is extremely difficult, regulation is dealt by comparing each one pair removing other plugs. When only one channel needs too strong stimulation, it is useful to regulate that pair after removing the plugs of other channels. By resetting the plug, stimulation control is often achieved. In that case, it must be paid attention to weaken the output of main controller for the sake of avoiding too strong stimulation by resetting the other plugs.
5. When the patient feels stimulation too strong at only one pair, we have to weaken the main controller so as to make the other points insensitive, controlling the most strongly felt part as it is adequate. Sometimes it is necessary to change the stimulation of that pair into retaining needle, moxa needle, acupoint injection or manipulation etc.

Best dose of stimulation is what the patient feels comfortable. It is extremely different person to person. The strength of adequate stimulation differs individually over 100 times as mentioned before.

C. Troubles of the Stimulator "Tokki"

If the patient does not feel any stimulation in spite of the strongest stimulation, some failure of instrument must be suspected.

Almost all the troubles of "Tokki" are distal from the channel as described below.

1) Wire Breakage

Most frequent mechanical trouble is wire breakage. It occurs at the connection point of plug or clip. Usually used Tokki (TypeⅢ) has voltmeter (not ammeter). Therefore, breakage cannot be recognized by voltmeter. So, dial indicator and instruments of soldering must be always ready.

2) Increase of Electric Resistivity of Indifferent Electrode Plate

Electric conductivity of indifferent electrode plate made of rubber degrades year by year. Then the patients' sensitivity seems to be lowered, or the patient feels prickling or tingling pain at indifferent plate. In such case, the plate must be renewed..

3) Faulty Setting of Plate

Faulty setting of indifferent electrode plate causes failure of stimulation.

There are causes as described below:

1. Electric cord comes off the plate.

    Because of the movement of patient (especially by getting up) sometimes electric cord comes off the plate. It is necessary to order patient not to get up after setting the plate.

2. Mistaking the Face of the Plate
Electrode plate has electric conductive face and non-conductive face. When stimulation is not felt in spite of strong output, it is necessary to check the mistake of setting plate.

3. Plate Does Not Contact Skin.
Sometimes plate is set on the undershirt. This is also to be checked when the stimulation is imperfect.

4) Mistake of Connecting Electric Cord
If the electric code of plate is connected with a anode, electric current does not run. When plug of electric code (which has its own color) is connected with wrong channel, stimulation control becomes difficult. By resetting after control with removing plug, attention is necessary not to mistake the position of the plug.

§ 3   Other Treatment with Filiform Needle (Body Acupuncture)

[1] Retaining Needle and Manipulation
When the treatment of more than 4 pairs of points is necessary, usually moxa needle is used for supplementation. If moxa needle is difficult to use, sometimes retaining needle is used. The method is mentioned before (p.98). In this case, it is the most important not to mistake the direction of insertion.

When rapid effects are expected except electro-acupuncture, manipulation as "burning mountain method" or "penetrating heaven cooling method" is used. Besides the case of "lack of channels", it is useful for correcting deterioration due to the error of supplementation & draining. Method is mentioned before (p.100&101).

[2] Moxa Needle
Moxa needle is a method to burn moxa at the handle of the inserted needle.

This method is invented by Mr. SASAGAWA Tomooki, and there is a minute operating manual of Mr. AKABANE Koubee.[21] But here only my method is mentioned.

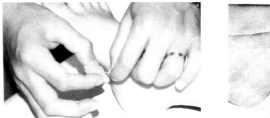 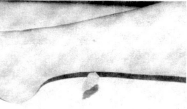

Fig.59   Moxa Needle

In my method, moxa needle is also used as a method of acupuncture therapy based on Meridian Theory, and meridian-and-point selection is quite the same as my electro-acupuncture. So, my method is considerably different from the operating manual of Mr. AKABANE [21].

Needle for this method has some necessary conditions. Handle of the needle must be made of metal. And the handle must not be soldered, but it must be welded or pressure bonded. In Japan "Needle for Moxa Needle" is put on the market.

Size of the needle for this method is No.20 (0.2mm in diameter) 5cm. Needles finer than No.20 are inadequate because they sag by the weight of moxa, and shorter needle is also inadequate because the moxa gets too close to the skin.

"Moxa for moxa needle" is also on the market. This is moxa of middle class quality. Moxa of top class quality is inadequate because it burns too rapidly, and moxa of inferior class is too fragile to set on the handle of needle. Recently carbonized smokeless moxa is available. But it seems not so convenient.

My method is different from Mr. AKABANE's method as mentioned below;

1) Direction of needle sticking

Needles are inserted not vertically but along the flow of the meridian, because this method is used for supplementation. But it must not be too oblique as retaining needle or electro-acupuncture, to avoid burning by radiant heat from the moxa.

2) Method of Setting Moxa

Dose of moxa is 0.3g to 0.5g for one needle. Moxa is stuck on the handle of the needle, compressed in the shape of conic or bullet form (because pointed tip is convenient for lighting fire). At this time, attention is necessary not to push the needle deeper into the skin. Mr. AKABANE's original method of moxa setting is to combine broken (into two pieces) moxa ball at the top of the handle of needle. For fear of unstable fixation of the moxa, this method is not used in my method.

3) Method to Light Moxa

For lightning moxa, lighter, matchlock or incense stick can be used. But match is not recommended for the fear if the head of match falls during burning.

There are two methods of lightning moxa, namely at the top and at the bottom. In my method, moxa is lighted at the top, because of the fear of the bearing capacity of ash of the moxa.

4) Shielding from Radiant Heat

Most of patient feels moxa needle comfortable. But radiant heat of moxa is fairly strong, and sometimes it is felt too hot. There is also a risk of burning. During moxa needle therapy, it is very important not to leave from the patient, and to ask the patient often if it is too hot. If the patient feels too hot, shielding wall made of paper is set for the protection from radiant heat. (Fig. 60)

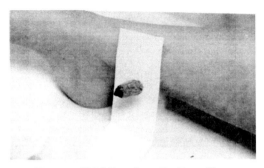

Fig.60 Shielding from Radiant Heat

Sometimes this paper shield is set ahead lightning moxa. If this shield is not effective, wet cotton (never use alcohol swab!) is put on the skin just under the burning moxa.

It is removed after the moxa become completely cool.

Heat sensetion by conductive heat rarely happens as far as the moxa is not too big, so as the burning moxa needle can be removed with fingers holding the needle body. So, generally, the effect of moxa needle is regarded to be the effect of radiant heat. Lightning at the bottom of moxa seems reasonable from this viewpoint.

However, in my method, when moxa is lighted at the tip, patient feels warm before radiant heat can reach the patient's skin. When the needle is inserted obliquely for a purpose of supplementation, heat source is not correctly above the acupuncture point, and radiant does not heat the point. Even so, excellent effects are obtained. Radiant heat shielding seems to give no influence for the effects

From these phenomena, the effect of conductive heat may not be neglected.

5) Method to Remove Ash of Moxa

Instrument for removing ash of moxa, a spoon with slit is available. But without such an instrument, ash is easily removed with two pieces of wet cotton (Fig.61).

Here attention should be paid to put appropriate pressure to the handle of the needle in order not to remove the needle.

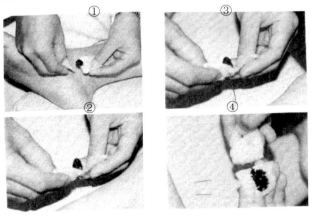

Fig.61 Removal of Ash of Moxa

6) Method of Needle Removal

After the removal of the ash, needles are removed as usual needle removal, usually slowly, with inspiration, and push the inserted point with swab because moxa needle treatment is used usually as supplementation.

7) Auxiliary Instruments

Besides the instrument for removing ash, cap with brim for moxa needle is available. But these instruments are not always necessary.

Attention by Moxa Needle

At the moxa needle treatment, the operator must be always careful about burn.

As the cause of burn, moxa dropping owing to mal-fixation or destruction of ash, radiant heat from moxa owing to too oblique stick or bending by fine needle or too much moxa and so on are enumerated. For the prevention of this accident, following attention must be paid.

1) Not to leave bed side of the patient until the moxa cools down.
2) Not to insert needle too obliquely.
3) Not to use too much moxa.
4) It is very important to confirm fixation of moxa.
5) Let the patient not move until moxa burns out and heat disappears.
6) Let the patient call out the operator **without moving body** whenever the patient feels hot.
7) Always be ready to fall of burning moxa or ash.
8) Disobedient patient, patient with involuntary movement or pathologic reflex is contraindication of moxa needle therapy.

Chapter 3 Other Acupuncture Therapies

§ 1 Intradermal Needle & Thumbtack Needle (cf. PART3)

Purpose of intradermal needle or thumbtack needle is as described below:
1) Prolongation of the effects.
2) Treatment of bronchial asthma or dermal diseases.
   For bronchial asthma, body acupuncture with filiform needle or acupoint injection etc. is very effective. Intradermal needle (including thumbtack needle) is also effective, and it prolongs the effect of body acupuncture. For dermal diseases, this therapy is often very effective singlehandedly. And it is also useful as supporting method for Kampo[Jp] medicine.
3) Treatment of joint pain.
4) When the treatment with filiform needle is difficult to use.

Intradermal needle is useful because it can be used both for supplementation and draining. In this case, attention should be paid for the direction (along or against the flow of the meridian) of needle insertion.

§ 2 Auricular Acupuncture [15)16)17)]

Auricular acupuncture is published by Dr. Paul NOGIER in 1957, that on the auricle there are reactive points corresponding to every part of the body, and many diseases and symptoms can be cured stimulating these points.

Many kinds of distribution maps of auricular points are published in China (Fig.62). Position of points is not always equal among charts, but according to any chart, good effects are obtained.

As target of auricular acupuncture, pain (especially pain of joints, tooth etc.), attack of asthma, symptoms concerning the inner ear as tinnitus or dizziness, symptoms of the eye or treatment of obesity etc. is listed. For the treatment of obesity, thumbtack needle is mainly used. For the treatment of the auricle with electro-acupuncture, short needle (20mm in length is best) is necessary.

Point is easily selected by searching distribution chart of auricular points. It is very easy, but points of ear are difficult to find neither by inspection nor by palpation. Usually they are searched by search meter or by pressure pain. Usually search meter is used, but detecting points by pressure pain with handle of needle or by stick pain is most easy and useful. The direction of sticking does not require careful consideration.

The auricle skin is closely adhered to cartilage except earlobe. Cartilage is very weak against infection. So, disinfection must be very strict like surgical operation, especially by retaining needle as the treatment of obesity.

120 PART 4 MY METHOD OF ACUPUNCTURE

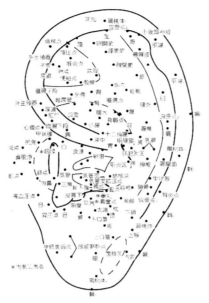

Fig.62 Points of Auricle
(According to "Ear Acupuncture" by Chinese Shanghai Military[17])

§ 3 Eyelid Acupuncture (p.183)

According to the late Mr. AOYAGI Seidou, a Japanese acupuncturist, there is relationship between the parts of eyelid and ORGANs, and treatment of each part produces effects for diseases or symptoms of correspondent ORGAN. In my method, this method is used only for the treatment of motor paralysis, together with body acupuncture, and it is occasionally very effective.

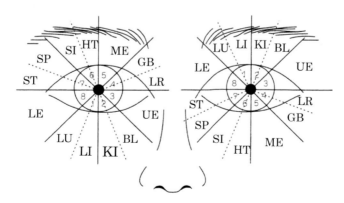

Fig.63 Relation between Eyelid and ORGANs

Chapter 3 Other Acupuncture Therapies 121

§ 4 SSP [6]

SSP can be called "acupuncture without puncture". This is corn shaped metal that can be used for electric stimulation. Usually it is applied symptomatically at the place of complaints. In my practice, it is used as an instrument for electric stimulation under the same principle of my electro-acupuncture, at the extremities, when needle insertion is not suitable. It is very convenient for the treatment of patients who has extraordinary feat for acupuncture or marked edema or hypersensitive reflex, and sometimes good effects are obtained. Compared with electro-acupuncture, much stronger stimulation is necessary and effect is evidently less.

Demerits of this method are:
1) This method is difficult to use at the head (haired part).
2) Control of supplementation and draining is difficult.
3) Hitting to correct point is difficult.
4) Correction of treatment error with manipulation is impossible.

From these factors, it may be difficult to make full use of this method for beginners.

§ 5 Acupoint Injection [22] (cf. p.v)

Acupuncture is a method of treatment inserting needle at some point, and giving some stimulation via the needle. If the acupuncture needle is replaced with injection needle and injection of some substance is given as stimulation, it is namely acupoint injection. So this method should be regarded as a kind of acupuncture. Here "injection itself" has the effect of acupuncture, and using pharmacologically quite inactive "medicine" as physiological saline solution or vitamins, excellent effects are obtained.

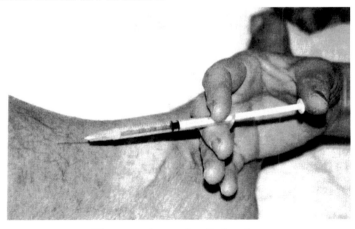

Fig.64 Acupoint Injection

This method is called "Point Injection" or "Water Acupuncture" in China, and "Pharmaco-(acu)puncture" in Korea, and extract of placenta or bee venom etc. are used as stimulating substances. This method is used in many countries. But the focus of argument seems the medicine to be used, and my logic seems not universal.

This method is far more simple and easier than other kind of acupuncture. Necessary instruments are only fine and rather long injection syringe of 1ml or 2ml and fine injection needle. Any substance that can be used subcutaneously or intramuscularly is usable. When pharmacologically active medicine is used, stronger and longer lasting effect is promptly obtained with less dose.

Principle of meridian selection and point selection is quite the same as electro-acupuncture in my method.

Method and Procedure of Practice

Meridians and points are selected according to the symptom or disease, and the injecting substance is selected according to the purpose. Method of injection is the same as intramuscular injection. Sensation of "Tokki" is rarely felt. If "Tokki" is felt, injection is done there. The depth of injection is usually half to 4/5 of the injection needle, but it is not definite. At the parts near bursa or joint, it is better to inject shallowly, like intradermal injection. When the injection hits good point, the patient sometimes feels as if something flows. But without this sensation, excellent effects are obtained.

Dose of injection is different according to the number of injecting points. Injection less than 0.03ml for one point can induce excellent effect.

Effects appear promptly, usually within several seconds. Severest pain as cancer pain can be sedated promptly by injection of analgesics or opiates to suitable points. Necessary dose is much less than usual use and the effect continues much longer.

Acupoint injection has the same merits as acupuncture, and its effects are almost the same as (sometimes better than) electro-acupuncture. Furthermore it is easier in the following points:

1) Consideration about Supplementation-or-Draining is not necessary.
   (Considering the condition, better effects are obtained.)
2) Fairly excellent effects are obtained as if needle does not hit points exactly.
3) Effects appear very rapidly, and propriety of points is immediately judged.
4) Many points can be treated simultaneously.
5) Everybody who is authorized to give injection can use this method easily.
   It is necessary to know meridian, but, for the time being, "try anyway seeing meridian chart!" is enough useful.

From the conditions 3) and 4), it is not necessary to worry about selection of meridian & point, and "trial of treatment one after another" is possible. And from this trial, order of points' importance is easily judged.

This method must be the easiest acupuncture.

§ 6　Finger Pressure to Acupuncture Points

The simplest method of point stimulation is finger pressure. It is only to strongly press points to be treated. Selection of meridians and points is the same as usual acupuncture of my method. Especially it is effective for headache, shoulder stiffness, lumber pain, dysmenorrhea and pollinosis. I have an experience of impressive case. The patient had severe lumber pain for several decades, and by finger pressure to BL_{60}, the pain disappeared promptly. I myself was quite astonished about the effect. If finger pressure is effective to any extent, acupuncture will be surely effective.

§ 7　Pasting Silver Grain or Magnetic Grain

This is a method to paste silver (silver gilded) grain of 1mm to 2mm in diameter or magnetic grain of several mm in diameter to points. Usually it is pasted at the place of complaints as symptomatic treatment. In my method, this method is used according to my policy of acupuncture, for the patient who hate acupuncture or at the place where infection is strongly worried as auricle. This method is rarely used, and the effect of this method is much lower than acupuncture. But sometimes unexpected effect appears. If this method is effective, the effect of acupuncture is surely expected.

There is other type of magnetic grain that has needle like thumbtack needle. But, as the risk of infection is not negligible, grain of this type is not recommended

Chapter 4   Appearance and Course of Effects

Type of appearance as well as the course of effect is various. Here the type by electro-acupuncture is explained, but type and course of effects are similar to that of other methods of acupuncture.

When the stimulation is adequate during the electro-acupuncture, moxa needle or retaining needle etc., the patient often falls asleep. And effects of such patients are almost always excellent.

Temporal course of effect is various as Fig 65. Type ⑤, ⑥ and ⑦ are most frequently observed. In these cases, sometimes effects appear at the next day. By many cases, effects appear just after the acupuncture or during acupuncture (Fig.64 ①, ②, ③,④).

In some cases complaints get worse after the acupuncture treatment (Fig.64 ⑫, ⑭). In such case, mistake of supplementation or draining should be reviewed at first. Many of them get better by correcting supplementation or draining. An impression is given that the patients who had some reaction, (getting better or worse) to acupuncture have possibility of effectiveness of acupuncture. Patients are laymen. With reverse effect, they assume that they got worse because of the acupuncture, losing trust in acupuncture. So, it is better to lessen the complaints immediately with manipulation or acupoint injection.

A few cases who got worse just after acupuncture and get better after a few days (Fig.64 ⑫). This may be a type of effect, but it cannot forecast at the time of treatment. Those who have no response (Fig.64 ⑬) or good effect for very short effect for long time are much more encouraging.

Most disappointing case is patients with no reaction (Fig.64 ⑬). In this case, the following factors are considered.
1) Correct chief complaints are not informed.
2) Strategy of meridian- &/or point- selection is mistaken.
3) Needle does not hit point exactly.
4) Case of delayed appearance of effects.
5) The case is not indication of acupuncture.

In these factors, case 5) is not so frequent, and 1), 2) and 3) should be well examined. If error was not found in these factors, it is worth while trying the same method about 10 times (at least 5 times). Not a few patients show some reaction during the trial. This phenomenon is very often observed by the treatment of post-herpetic neuralgia. Especially in case of severest pain, it is rather usual.

There are often some relation between the course of effects and diseases.

Type ③ and ④ appear in many cases, especially by treatment of whiplash syndrome in early stage. Practitioners feel disappointed by this type, especially when this type continues for long time. Many cases of this type, effects last longer while continuing treatment, changing into type ②.

In the effects type ④ which continue very long time, sometimes it is caused by cancer pain or diabetic neuralgia. If this type continues long time (over a few weeks or more), the patient is recommend to have a medical checking.

Rebound (type ⑧) appears very often by fresh Herpes Zoster. In spite of excellent effect, pain with fresh Herpes Zoster reappears after 30minutes to 3hours after the treatment. Often the patient feels stronger pain than before the treatment, and it hurts patient's confidence to acupuncture so much. It is very important to explain the course of effect before the treatment. This phenomenon appears (although not so frequent) when the stimulation is too strong or too long in other diseases or symptoms.

Type ⑩ and ⑪ sometimes appear, but the relation between diseases is not clear. For the present, the effect is valued "ineffective" when the effect does not appear within 2days. But I have an experience of one patient who had lumber pain for over several years, completely cured with one time acupuncture treatment, although the effect appeared about one week after the treatment.

Type ⑫ and ⑭ are not yet experienced.

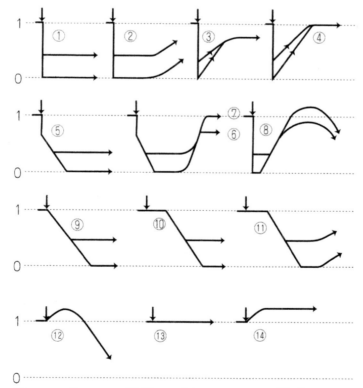

Fig.65 Course of Effect of Acupuncture Therapy

PART 5
COMPLICATIONS, SIDE EFFECTS & CASES OUT OF ACUPUNCTURE

Chapter 1 Complications and Side Effects of Acupuncture

As the complications and the side effects of acupuncture, bleeding, needle breakage, infection, pneumothorax, burn by moxa needle, so called cerebral anemia and aggravation of symptoms are listed in the textbooks of acupuncture. In these complications and side effects, most of aggravation would be due to mistake of supplementation and draining. Pneumothorax cannot happen in my practice. So called cerebral anemia will seldom happen by supine position. I have not yet experienced it. Burn by moxa needle is nothing but careless mistake. Bleeding and pain by needle puncture are unavoidable. But it is usually not serious.

As complications of acupuncture in my practice, pain, bleeding, needle breakage and infection may be enumerated. I have not yet experienced "side effects".

§ 1 Leaving Needle

"Left needle after the treatment" is one of careless mistakes of acupuncture. Usually it is soon noticed, but occasionally needle is carelessly left for long time. Actually, harm by this mistake is not frequent. But possibility of infection cannot be neglected, and confidence of patient and reputation can be highly hurt.

Head, especially in the hair, and hardly visible parts must be most careful. To avoid this mistake, it is recommended to remove needles symmetrically one by one especially at such places.

§ 2 Bleeding

Small venous bleeding is unavoidable but harmless. Large bleeding due to sticking artery is theoretically possible, but I have no experience of this event. Fine artery will avoid itself from needle, and when the needle hits not fine artery, the practitioner will feel pulsation of the artery and he will not dare to push the needle more. If fine needle of 0.2mm in diameter or so penetrated artery, pushing the penetrated part for several minutes, hematoma-forming will be prevented completely (except patients of hemophilia).

By acupoint injection, as needle is relatively thick, risk of bleeding is somewhat larger. I have no experience of sticking artery, but if the needle sticks artery, it will be promptly realized by back current of blood. By prompt removing needle and pushing the part for several minutes forming hematoma will be prevented.

It is impossible never to hurt blood vessel by acupuncture. So, it is impossible to prevent bleeding completely. It is very important to explain that bleeding is unavoidable and that the bruise according to bleeding surely disappears and it is no need to worry. It is to be paid attention to avoid sticking needle at noticeable parts as the face.

Sometimes point situates just on a vein. The method to avoid stick the vein is to insert needle without needle tube at the edge of the vein, and aim the deep point. It is not easy for beginners.

If the needle tip is damaged, not only the patient feels pain but also the risk of bleeding increases. By use of disposable needle this risk is negligible.

§ 3   Needle Breakage

Acupuncture needle is very fine. Broken needle is clearly visible on the X-ray film, but on the image intensifier it can hardly recognized. So, it is extremely difficult to remove broken acupuncture needle. I have some experiences of extirpation of remained broken acupuncture needle. It was extremely strenuous to find the needle. The most serious complication of acupuncture may be needle breakage.

Quality of recent Japanese filiform needle is excellent, and it is scarcely broken. By use of disposable needle, metal fatigue is out of anxiety. But by repeating use of needle, enough attention must be paid for metal fatigue. Metal fatigue is apt to happen at bent potion. So, bent needle must never be used. Bent portion is easily found by palpating needle with fingers. "Bent needle should be scraped". This is the most simple and sure method to avoid needle breakage by metal fatigue.

Electrolysis happens at anode. Stimulation of most electric stimulator is bipolar spike wave. Thereby electric current is passed between needle and needle. I am afraid if electrolysis would happen at anode phase of stimulation. Stimulation of "Tokki" is given only by cathode rectangular wave. So it may be very safe for electrolysis.

Anyway, by electric stimulation, needles less than 0.2mm in diameter are inadequate. When stimulation for a very long time is necessary as acupuncture anesthesia, dicker needle should be used.

§ 4   Infection

Attention to infection was rather insufficient until recently in the world of acupuncture.

Skin has a strong barrier against bacterial infection.

The tissue of the skin has tight heap of collagen fibers, and pyogenic bacteria are captured within shallow layer of the skin being wiped by collagen fiber during needle passes this layer. Infection in the shape of suppuration may have been seldom owing to this barrier. But this "barrier" is powerless against virus. Now attention to infection must be paid more seriously.

Infection is formed by following three factors:

1) Invasion of pyogenic microbes into the body (Contamination).
2) Multiplication of microbes in the body.
3) Bad influence for the body by the multiplication of pyogenic microbes.

There are many methods to overcome these factors. But without contamination, infection never appears. So, the most simple and sure method to prevent infection is to avoid contamination.

As the cause of contamination by acupuncture, imperfect disinfection of skin and contamination of needle body is enumerated.

[1] Contamination due to Imperfect Disinfection of the Skin

A. Dirty Skin

The first step of disinfection is to mechanically remove dirt of the operation field. The field must be kept at least "dirt is not visible on the used alcohol swab". Sometimes this factor seems to be made light.

B. Unsuitable Disinfectants

In usual cases, disinfection with alcohol swab is enough useful as usual injection. But there are weak parts against infection as auricle. There disinfection must be stronger. For such places, alcohol swab is used as skin cleaning, and thereafter disinfection with stronger disinfectants as povidone iodine must be used.

C. Contaminated Disinfectants

Effect of disinfectants is not always perfect. If the disinfectant itself is contaminated, the "disinfection" cannot be enough effective.

Followings can be the cause.

1) Imperfect disinfection of cotton swab
2) Contamination from practitioner's finger
3) Contamination from the patient's skin
4) Contamination from the aseptic itself

1) Imperfect disinfection of cotton swab

Alcohol swab made of commercially available cotton may be practically useful as it is used for injection. But considering the sterilizing effect of alcohol, it may be better to use sterilized cotton.

2) Contamination from fingers of the practitioner

When the practitioner's fingers are not clean, the dirt can be transmitted into the skin. Cleanness of the fingers must be always paid attention, not to say as clean as by surgical operation.

"Once disinfected parts" should not be touched with practitioner's finger as if the finger is clean in usual meaning. The most simple and surest method is "needle body where it can enter the body must not be touched with the fingers".

3) Contamination from the patient's skin

Sometimes wound or inflammation is found near the point. "Disinfection" with swab which passed that place can contaminate the field. It is better not to use such point, but treatment of the point is necessary by all means, effort must be made not to contaminate the field considering the direction of cleaning.

"Disinfect many parts with one swab" is not recommended. "One swab for one part" is sometimes insufficient. If the swab is found not clean at the first "disinfection", this "disinfection" should be regarded as cleaning, and with second swab, "real disinfection" should be given.

4) Contamination of disinfectant itself

Disinfectant in a contaminated bottle is not clean. If too much alcohol of cotton swab is squeezed into the bottle, everything in the bottle is contaminated by the dirt of from fingers. It should be strictly prohibited.

[2] Contamination by Contaminated Needle Body

This type of contamination is composed of imperfect disinfection of needle and improper use of needle.

A. Contamination by Imperfect Disinfection of Needle

Not "disinfected" but "sterilized" needle is desirable. Repeatedly used needle is better to be sterilized by autoclaving. Using disposable needle, this problem is easily cleared up. But by disposable needle without stopper, although rarely, owing to deficiency of stopping function, needle moves during transportation. Attention must be paid about this type of contamination.

B. Contamination due to Improper Use of Needle

As if needle is perfectly sterilized, the needle becomes contaminated at the time of insertion by improper aseptic technique of the operator. To avoid this contamination, it is necessary that "the part of needle body which will enter into the body must be kept clean". That is, "the part which can enter into the body must not be touched with bacteriologically dirty matters". Here, most attention must be paid for "indirect contamination". "Things that have contacted dirty matter becomes dirty" is common sense of surgeon.

In acupuncture treatment, practitioner'sfingers are far from the aseptic state, even if well washed and "disinfected". And the field of acupuncture cannot be kept clean as surgical operation field. This circumstance must be always kept in mind. "Licking needle before insertion" or "insertion through clothes" as in remote past days is an extreme example. I would like to believe that there are no such cases nowadays.

1) Contamination through needle tube

When needle passes needle tube, tip of the needle certainly touches the wall of needle tube. By use of repeatedly using needle tube, pollution of wall of needle tube (by contaminated handle of needle) becomes worse in every each use. To avoid this contamination completely, there is no other choice than to use disposable needle with needle tube or to insert needle without needle tube.

2) Contamination by Needle Sticking and Insertion

If contaminated needle is inserted into the body, it is evidently contamination. Practitioner's fingers are not sterile. Even if they are well disinfected, it is difficult to keep them sterile. Part of needle body that touched practitioner's finger should be regarded to be contaminated.

The technique to insert needle without touching needle body (which can enter into the skin) is explained before (Part3 Chapter1 p.91, 92).

3) Contamination in Needle Case

Sterilized or disinfected needles are stored by many methods. A method is often used to keep scores of needles in one case for disinfection (or sterilization) and the case is stored in clean state. The method itself is not unsuitable if the state of storage is dry, and needle is picked out one by one with dry sterile forceps. But if a needle is picked out with fingers, especially needles are wet, all needles in the "disinfected" case can be contaminated by the stain of the operator's fingers.

Recently sterilized disposable needle is mainly used. In the circumstance that disposable needle is not available, it is recommended to sterilize needles by autoclave or gas sterilization, and to pack needles in suitable number, as one pair or subset of 6 needles. By this method, needles can be picked up with "not clean" fingers without contamination.

§ 5   Side Effects of Acupuncture

Pain by needle puncture is unavoidable. This may be minute "side effect" of acupuncture. There are some kinds of painless acupuncture as subcutaneous acupuncture, thumbtack needle or very shallow puncture of filiform needle etc. that produces fairly excellent effects. But, in my impression, deeper insertion with "Tokki$^{(Jp.)}$ (Gettiing K$^{(Jp.)}$I(QI$^{(Ch.)}$))" causes better effects.

In many textbooks, so called "cerebral anemia" is listed as side effect. But I have no experience of this "side effect". It may be very rare by supine position.

Deterioration of symptoms is often listed as side effect of acupuncture. But, in my experience, most of them seem due to mistake of supplementation and draining, and deterioration is easily corrected by correcting the method of supplementation and draining. This may be called rather "medical error". But this error scarcely brings serious consequence as medical errors of Occidental Medicine.

Sometimes pain or numbness remains at the treated part. Usually it disappears in several days. If the treatment demands extremely long time, it is better not to use same points too frequently.

Bathing after acupuncture or overwork on the next day occasionally causes heavy fatigue. Guidance for patients about these "side effects" is necessary.

Chapter 2 Diseases out of Indication & Contraindications of Acupuncture

§ 1 Diseases out of Indication of Acupuncture [23]

As though acupuncture has vast range of indication, it is not almighty. Followings are listed as out of indication in textbooks.

Tumors	Aortic aneurythma
Temporal arteritis	Obstructive arterial diseases
Tuberculosis	Subdural hematoma
Vertebral disc hernia	Hunt Syndrome
Sudden deafness	Ossifying tendinitis
Spinocerebellar degeneration	Fracture
Amyotrophic lateral sclerosis	Medial meniscus injury
Ileus	Myocardial infarction
Urinary calculus	Angina pectoris
Uterine myoma	

Ossification of posterior longitudinal ligament of vertebra   etc.

Among these diseases, most of Hunt Syndrome can be cured by acupuncture. Pain of vertebral disc hernia or spinal canal stenosis is often markedly diminishes, sometimes the complaints completely vanish by acupuncture therapy. But for most of above mentioned diseases, it is reckless to attempt to "cure" with acupuncture.

There are many other diseases which cannot be cured by acupuncture. However, it does not mean that these diseases are completely out of indication of acupuncture.

It is sure that acupuncture should not want to "cure" diseases for which Occidental Medicine has established method of treatment, except those which acupuncture is evidently effective as Herpes Zoster, bronchial asthma, pollinosis, dysmenorrhea or whiplash syndrome etc. But this does not mean that acupuncture should never be used for these diseases. Even if those diseases have no method to be treated by Occidental Medicine or in addition to Occidental therapy, acupuncture is surely useful. "Acupuncture for relieving complaints" is very meaningful. "Acupuncture cannot be main treatment = Contraindication of acupuncture" must be also a mistake

§ 2 Cases out of Indication of Electro-acupuncture

My method of electro-acupuncture is difficult to apply following cases.

1) Children

2) Those Who Cannot Respond

In my method, "balance taking" is essentially important. So, without accurate answer, good treatment is impossible. Followings are such cases.

  1. Deafness, aphasia, or heavy dysphasia
  2. Heavy dementia
  3. Those who cannot take communication (such as foreigners etc.)

3) Treatment at Anesthetized Part

Even by patients of cerebrovascular diseases who have sensory disturbances, effects of electro-acupuncture are expected so long as the patient can feel stimulation. But, acupuncture is ineffective at the completely anesthetized part such as patients of spinal injury. Also acupoint injection cannot cause any effect better than pharmacological effects for these cases.

4) Those Who Have Abnormal Movements

If the patient has involuntary movement, needle insertion itself is difficult. As if needle puncture is achieved, needle bending often appears and risk of needle breakage is not negligible. Such cases must be regarded as contraindication of treatment with filiform needle.

In patients with pathological reflex as cerebrospinal vascular diseases, strong reflex movement can happen by slightest stimulation. Even stimulation at the "safe part" can induce strong reflex at other parts. For these patients, moxa needle is also difficult to use.

Some patients move hand with answer for question. In patients with low ability of understanding, often this action cannot be inhibited. For these patient, acupuncture at upper extremity is difficult. Acupuncture as well as moxa needle may be regarded as contraindication for these patients.

5) Those Who Have Electronic Items (like cardic pasemaker) in the Body.

§ 3 Contraindication of Intradermal acupuncture & Thumbtack Needle

Intradermal acupuncture and thumbtack needle are almost painless and good (often excellent) effects are expected. However, these needles have a risk of unconscious falling. When the patient lives with babies or infants, the risk of swallowing the lost needle is not negligible. Those patient who have small children must be regarded as contraindication of all kind of intradermal acupuncture.

§ 4   Contraindication of Acupuncture

There are "Acupuncture Forbidden Points". They are the points which are regarded to be risky to insert. For example, GV_{15} (medulla oblongata), LI_{13} (radial nerve) or GB_3 (vessels) etc. are enumerated.

SP_6 is also listed as the acupuncture prohibited point for pregnant person, because of the risk of abortion. But, recently, this point is often used for the treatment of breech.

There are points at breast, back or supraclavicular fossa which have risk of pneumothorax. But they are not always prohibited according to the method of use. In my practice, these dangerous region is never used for acupuncture. So, there is no need to worry about pneumothorax.

It should be prohibited to give acupuncture at the part of dermal diseases, especially at the part of infection. And it may be better to avoid insert needle at the place with strong edema.

Otherwise there may not be any cases that are prohibited to treat with acupuncture by any method.

PART 6   PRACTICE OF ACUPUNCTURE

Chapter 1   Pain (Including Stiffness & Numbness)

§ 1   General Rule

Method of treatment for stiffness and numbness is the same as treatment of pain. Effects for numbness are often inferior to pain. Electro-acupuncture and acupoint injection are most often used, and moxa needle is also used together with electro-acupuncture. For severest pain, acupoint injection with analgesics is very useful. It is also useful for meridian-&-point selection when the practitioner worries about it. Thumbtack needle or intradermal acupuncture is useful as supporting use of acupuncture, and sometimes they are used as the main treatment.

Principle of meridian selection for pain is to select meridians that pass through the area of the pain as mentioned before (PART 2). It is effective almost without exception. There, classic meridians which are not illustrated in general meridian charts are sometimes very important.

The most important factor by meridian selection is to confirm the localization of pain exactly as mentioned before (PART 2 and PART 4). If it is not correct, good effect is never obtained. Any point on the suitable meridian can be used regardless of function of the points. Usually, points that are easy to use are selected.

Effect is excellent. Process of effect is not uniform according to the cause of the disease or the method of treatment. Appearance of effect is very rapid by acupoint injection. Whereas effect of electro-acupuncture often appears a little later, but its effect is mostly better and longer lasting.

The principle of the treatment of pain is the fundamental principle of my method. This principle can be applied for many other complaints.

In following cases, effect of the acupuncture is (sometimes apparently) not clear.

1) Patients with Sensory Paralysis

Acupuncture at anesthetic part is ineffective. By such case, acupuncture must be given at sensory sound parts as the trunk or the head.

2) Post-herpetic Neuralgia (PHN)

Many patients of PHN do not feel effect after the treatment subjectively, as if the effect is objectively marked. This phenomenon will be mentioned later.

3) Pain Caused by Injury of Central Nerve

In acupoint injection with Pentazocine or opiates, almost all kinds of pain, such as severest cancer pain, can be sedated. However, in my experiences, good effect was not obtained for the patient of thalamic pain or the pain caused injury of the spinal cord. My method may not be indication of that kind of pain.

4) Fresh Injury

Electro-acupuncture is difficult to use for fresh injury except compression fracture of vertebra. There, acupoint injection with analgesics is mainly used if necessary.

5) Pain Caused by Excessive Deformity

For the pain which is caused by high grade deformity, acupuncture is often ineffective, or, as if it is effective for a while, its duration is often short.

6) Psychogenic Pain

Among patients of whiplash syndrome, although fairly rare, some cases show unexpectedly insufficient effect. One type is effect itself is insufficient (this type is rare), and the other is "good but short lasting" effect continues for a long time. Almost all patients have no unreasonable symptoms. But some of such patients do not come after settlement of compensation. It is uncertain if this is malingering or no, but the pain of such patient may be strongly affected by psychogenic factor.

Principle of acupuncture therapy for pain has many common points with the treatment of other diseases or symptoms. At the start of acupuncture therapy, comprehension of this chapter will be surely helpful.

§ 2   Head (Except Face)

Pain in the head and/or the face is one of the best indications of acupuncture.

There are numerous causes of headache including obscure origin as general malaise, postmenopausal syndrome or autonomic ataxia etc. Symptomatic headache such as brain tumor, intracranial hematoma, temporal arteritis, meningitis or glaucoma etc. is absolute indication of Occidental Medicine, and they should be excluded from the indication of acupuncture (except as supportive treatment). But the patients suffering from functional headache (which occupies from 70% to 80% of headache) expect only to sedate the pain even in Occidental Medicine. For such cases acupuncture is very useful. And the strategy of treatment is, regardless of the cause of the pain, with the same pattern according to the location of the pain.

Point selection is only to select on the meridians that pass through the part of the pain as described below. The meridians to be treated are:

1. Around the center line of the nape, occipital region, parietal region, around center of the forehead or the zone including them.
2. Outer side of the nape, temporal to parietal region, outer side of the forehead or the part including them.
3. Posterolateral side of the neck, temporal to retro-auricular region, the temple or the range including them.
4. Forehead
5. Broad area or obscure region

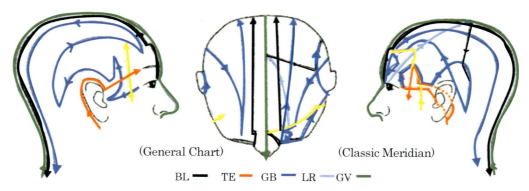

Fig.66 Meridians of head

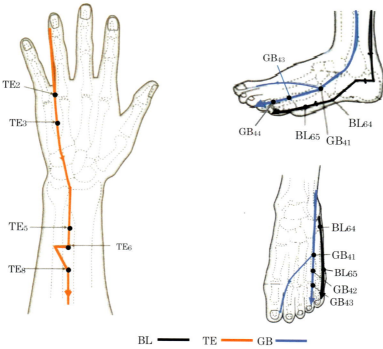

Fig.67 Points for Treatment of Headache

[1] Around the Center Line

Here the leading role is BLADDER Meridian (BL). With electro-acupuncture, BL_{64} is most useful. By acupoint injection, BL_{60}, BL_{61}, BL_{62} BL_{64}, or BL_{65} are used taking the effect into account. Using the points of GALLBLADDER Meridian as GB_{41}, GB_{42} or GB_{43} etc. together, effects are often markedly intensified.

[2] Outer Side of the Center Line to Parietal Region

Here the leading role is GALLBLADDER Meridian (GB). GB_{41}, G_{42} or GB_{43} is most often used by electro-acupuncture. Using the points of BLADDER Meridian (BL) such as BL$_{64}$ or BL$_{65}$ etc. and the points of TRIPLE ENERGIZER Meridian (TE) such as TE$_2$, TE$_3$ or TE$_5$ together, effects are often markedly intensified.

[3] **Temporal- & Retro-auricular Region, Temple & Lateral Neck**

Here the leading role is TRIPLE ENERGIZER Meridian (TE). TE$_2$, TE$_3$, TE$_5$ and TE$_8$ are most frequently used. Using points of GALLBLADDER Meridian (GB) such as GB$_{41}$, GB$_{42}$ or GB$_{43}$ etc. together, effects are often markedly intensified.

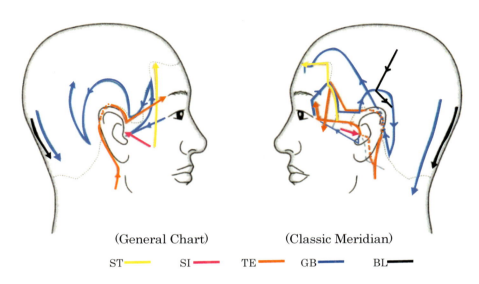

(General Chart)   (Classic Meridian)

ST——   SI——   TE——   GB——   BL——

Fig.68   Meridians of Temporal & Retro-auricular Area

[4] **Forehead and Lateral Part of the Forehead**

Mainly points of GALLBLADDER MERIDIAN (GB$_{41}$, GB$_{42}$ or GB$_{43}$ etc.) and TRIPLE ENERGIZER Meridian (TE$_3$, TE$_5$ or TE$_8$ etc.) are used for the pain in this area. If effects are not enough, using the points of STOMACH Meridian (ST$_{43}$, ST$_{44}$ etc.) concurrently, often good effect is obtained. Sometimes excluding point on STOMACH Meridian, treatment is not effective.

[5] **Pain at Broad Area or Obscure Region**

In this case, treatment of points of BLADDER(BL)-, TRIPLE ENERGIZER(TE)- and GALLBLADDER(GB)- Meridian are used. Combination of BL$_{64}$, TE$_5$ and GB$_{41}$ is most convenient to use. If forehead is contained, it is better to add the point of STOMACH Meridian such as ST$_{43}$ or ST$_{44}$. To detect most important point (or meridian), acupoint injection is useful. Using bilateral injection, the most important point becomes clear automatically.

138   PART 6   PRACTICE OF ACUPUNCTURE

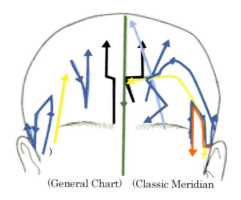

Fig. 69-1   Meridians of Forehead

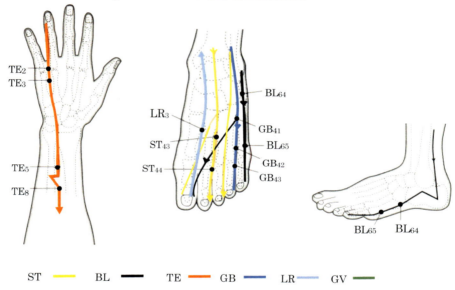

Fig. 69-2   Points for Headache of Forehead

§ 3   Face and Mouth

As the targets of this area, toothache, series of the pain at the region of trigeminal nerve (idiopathic trigeminal neuralgia, atypical facial pain, cluster headache etc.), Herpes Zoster, tumor pain, troubles of the eye and intraoral pain are listed. For all these events, acupuncture can be applied by the same pattern with excellent effect.

Acupoint injection is also effective in the same way. Any substance (for subcutaneous or intramuscular injection) can be used with excellent effect, but for the severe pain such as cancer pain, analgesic agents or opiates are necessary.

[1] Eye

In general meridian charts, no meridian neither passes nor enters into the eye.

According to the classic literatures, distribution of meridians around eye is like Fig.70. Among these meridians, LIVER Meridian (LR) passes the eye, and CONCEPTION VESSEL (CV) enters into the eye. And HEART Meridian (HT) and GALLBLADDER Meridian (GB) reach the eye.

For most of complaints of the eye can be resolved by treatment of LR$_3$. By treatment of HEART Meridian (HT) or GALLBLADDER Meridian (GB), patients often tell that view became clearer. Points of these meridians are also useful for the complaints of the eye. But these points are seldom used because treatment of LR$_3$ is almost 100% effective.

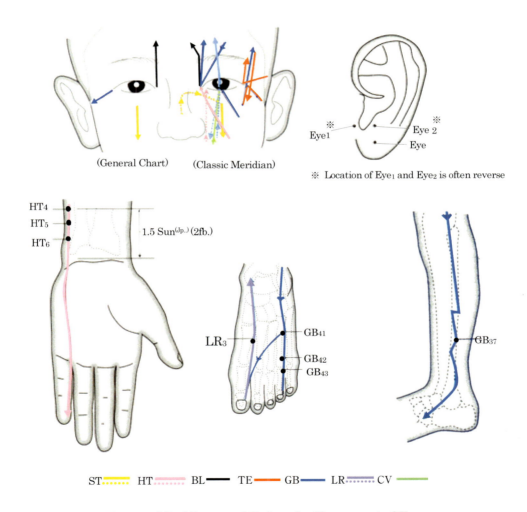

Fig.70 Meridians and Points for Treatment of Eye

[2] Toothache

Many meridians pass through the upper- and the lower- jaw as Fig.71. But only LARGE INTESTINE Meridian (LI) and STOMACH Meridian (ST) are described to "enter into the teeth". For many cases, treatment of only LI$_4$ is enough effective. If the effect is insufficient, adding treatment of the points of STOMACH Meridian (ST$_{43}$, ST$_{44}$ etc.), better effect is obtained. For most cases, acupoint injection is effective. Usually it is not necessary to use analgesic agents. Treatment of "point of anesthesia for tooth extraction" of the ear is also very effective. Auricular acupuncture is useful when the treatment of body acupuncture (including acupoint injection) is not enough effective.

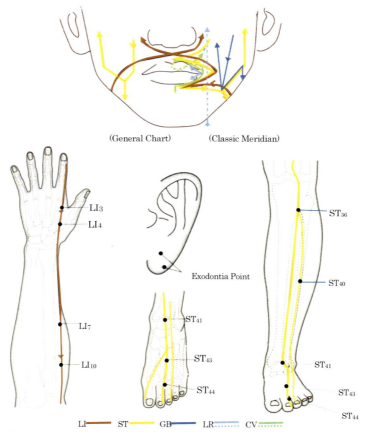

Fig.71 Meridians Related with Teeth and Points for Treatment of Toothache

[3] Oral Cavity and/or Tongue

SPLEEN Meridian (SP) spreads under the tongue, and one branch of LIVER Meridian (LR) passes around inner side of the cheek and the lip. For the complaints of this area, treatment of SP$_3$ or SP$_4$ is effective. Sometimes the pain is sedated by only shallow needle puncture such as thumbtack needle. Acupoint injection is also effective.

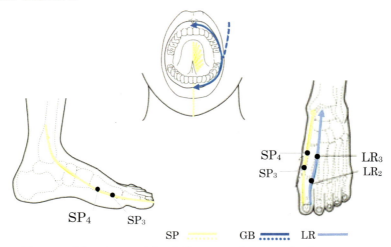

Fig.72　Meridians of Oral Cavity and Points for Treatment

[4] Throat

According to the classic literatures, SPLEEN Meridian (SP), HEART Meridian (HT), KIDNEY Meridian (KI) and LIVER Meridian (LR) pass through the area of the trachea and the throat.

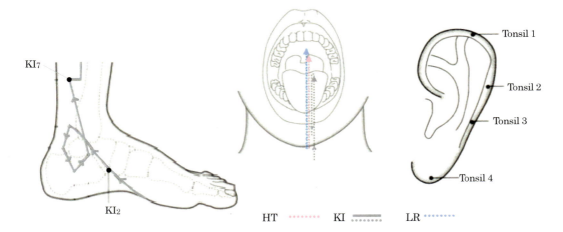

Fig.73　Meridians of Throat and Points for Treatment

142 PART 6 PRACTICE OF ACUPUNCTURE

Some Kampo formulas are very effective for the inflammation of the throat. Acupuncture is also effective, and its effect appears promptly. Mainly the points on KIDNEY Meridian is used. There are several opinions about the direction of flow of this meridian from KI$_2$ to KI$_7$, and direction of flow of the meridian is hardly decided. So, mainly KI$_2$ is used for body acupuncture. By acupoint injection, other points on KIDNEY Meridian can be used. Points of auricle are seldom used.

[5] Face
1) Lower Jaw

Many meridians pass through this area. However, treatment of STOMACH Meridian (ST$_{41}$, ST$_{43}$, ST$_{44}$ etc.) is effective for almost all the cases. Treatment of LARGE INTESTINE Meridian (LI$_3$, LI$_4$ etc.) is also effective.

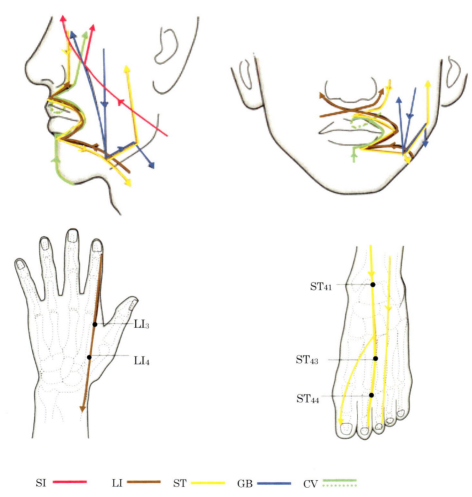

Fig.74 Meridians and Points for Treatment of Lower Jaw

2) Upper Jaw & Zygomatic Region

According to the classic literatures, many meridians pass through this area.

The most common target at upper jaw is toothache. For any kind of pain, treatment of LARGE INTESTINE Meridian (mainly LI$_4$) and sometimes with STOMACH Meridian (ST$_{43}$, ST$_{44}$ etc.) is effective.

Most of the pain at the zygomatic region can be sedated by the treatment of points of SMALL INTESTINE Meridian (SI$_3$ or SI$_4$, and acupoint injection to SI$_6$). Sometimes using together with points of STOMACH Meridian (ST$_{43}$, ST$_{44}$ etc.) and/or GALLBLADDER Meridian (GB$_{41}$, GB$_{42}$ or GB$_{43}$ etc.) promotes the effect.

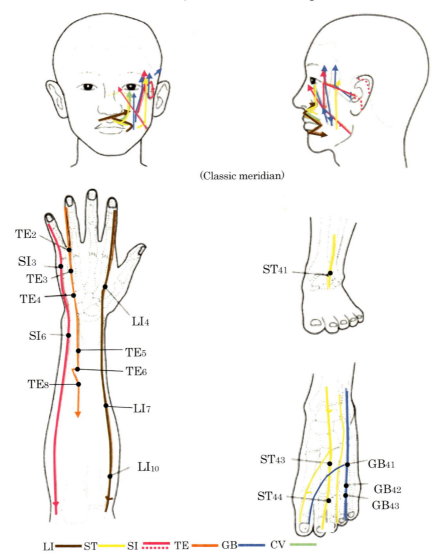

Fig.75 Meridians & Points for Treatment of Upper Jaw & Zygomatic Region

3) Around the Nose

In general charts, only GOVERNOR VESSEL (GV) and LARGE INTESTINE Meridian (LI) are illustrated around the nose. But according to the classic literatures, STOMACH Meridian (ST) starts from the bridge of the nose. Points of LARGE INTESTINE Meridian (LI_3, LI_4, LI_{10} etc.) and/or STOMACH Meridian (ST_{36}, ST_{43}, ST_{44} etc.) are used for complaints of the nose with excellent effects. Sometimes treatment of points of BLADDER Meridian (BL64, BL65 etc.,) is effective for the complaint of the nose.

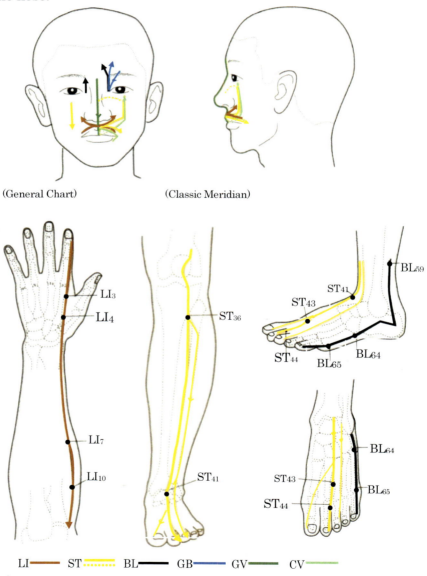

Fig.76 Meridians & Points for Treatment of Nose-Area

4) Forehead

In general meridian charts, GOVERNOR VESSEL (GV), BLADDER Meridian (BL), GALLBLADDER Meridian (GB) and STOMACH Meridian (ST) are illustrated. According to the classic literatures, STOMACH Meridian (ST) passes along the total hairline of the forehead, and TRIPLE ENERGIZER Meridian (TE) and LIVER Meridian (LR) also pass here. But their pathways in charts are not always the same.

For the treatment of the forehead, points of TRIPLE ENERGIZER Meridian (TE$_2$, TE$_3$, TE$_5$ or TE$_8$), GALLBLADDER Meridian (GB$_{41}$, GB$_{42}$ or GB$_{43}$) and/or STOMACH Meridian (ST$_{43}$ or ST$_{44}$) are treated. If the pain is localized around hairline, treatment of STOMACH Meridian (ST) is especially effective.

Acupoint injection is very useful for detecting effective points.

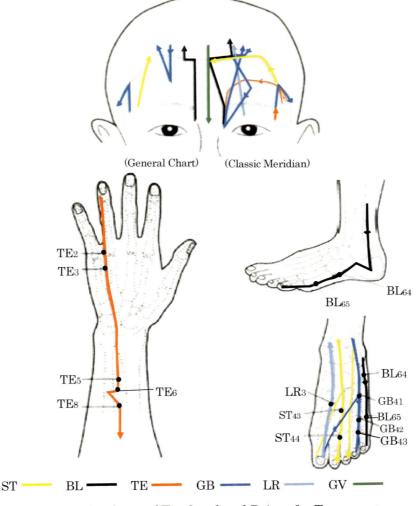

Fig.77 Meridians of Forehead and Points for Treatment

146 PART 6 PRACTICE OF ACUPUNCTURE

§ 4　Neck

[1] Back of the Neck (Fig.78)

Pain and/or stiffness of this area is one of the most frequently complained symptom together with headache &/or shoulder stiffness, and it is a good indication of acupuncture. In general meridian charts, GOVERNOR VESSEL (GV), BLADDER Meridian (BL) and GALLBLADDER Meridian (GB) pass through this area, but according to the classic literatures, TRIPLE ENERGIZER Meridian (TE) also passes here.

Almost all cases of pain (&/or stiffness) of this area can be cured by treating points of BLADDER Meridian (BL_{64} or BL_{65}) and GALLBLADDER Meridian (GB_{41}, GB_{42} or GB_{43}). If the effect is insufficient, acupoint injection to GV_{14} is effective.

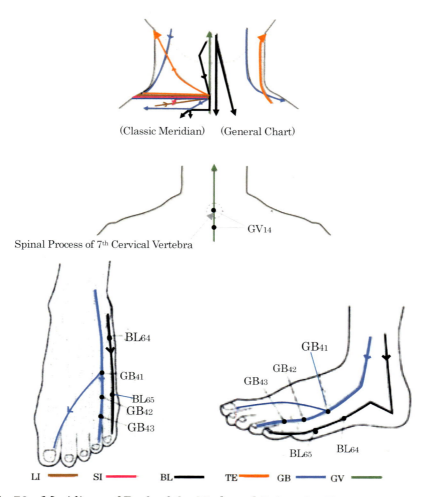

Fig.78　Meridians of Back of the Neck and Points for Treatment

[2] Anterior &/or Lateral Part of the Neck (Fig.76)

In general meridian charts, CONCEPTION VESSEL (CV), STOMACH Meridian (ST), LARGE INTESTINE Meridian (LI) and SMALL INTESTINE Meridian (SI) are illustrated. According to the classic literatures, also SPLEEN Meridian (SP), HEART Meridian (HT), KIDNEY Meridian (KI), GALLBLADDER Meridian (GB) and LIVER Meridian (LR) pass through this area, but their pathways are not clear.

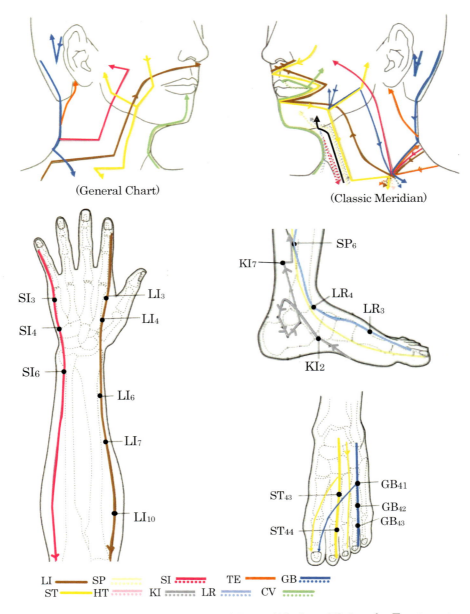

Fig.79 Meridians of Anterior- to Lateral Part of Neck and Points for Treatment

LARGE INTESTINE Meridian (mostly LI$_4$, sometimes LI$_3$, LI$_6$, LI$_7$ or LI$_{10}$) and SMALL INTESTINE Meridian (SI$_3$ or SI$_4$), and SI$_6$ (for acupoint injection) are used with excellent effects.

For the pain of the anterior neck, mainly points of LARGE INTESTINE Meridian (mainly LI$_4$) and STOMACH Meridian (ST$_{43}$, ST$_{44}$ etc.) are used with excellent effects. In some cases, points of SPLEEN Meridian (SP$_3$, SP$_4$ etc.), KIDNEY Meridian (KI$_2$, KI$_7$ etc.) &/or LIVER Meridin(mainly LR$_3$) are used. About KIDNEY Meridian, KI$_3$, KI$_4$, KI$_5$ or KI$_6$ etc. are also used for acupoint injection and thumbtack needle.

For the treatment of pain at the lateral neck, Points of LARGE INTESTINE Meridian (mostly LI$_4$, sometimes LI$_3$, LI$_6$, LI$_7$ or LI$_{10}$) and SMALL INTESTINE Meridian (SI$_3$ or SI$_4$, and SI$_6$ (for acupoint injection) are used with excellent effects.

§ 5 "Shoulder" & Shoulder Joint

"Pain of shoulder" does not always mean "pain of the shoulder joint". Region from anterior edge of the trapezius muscle to the scapular body is widely called "shoulder", and most of "shoulder stiffness" is stiff feeling of this area. This area is called "Shoulder" in this book. "Range of the shoulder" of patients is very wide. For example, the shoulder means back of the neck for someone, the interscapular region, and even the upper part of the arm for someone. So it is very important to confirm the "place of shoulder" strictly before treatment.

[1] "Shoulder"

LARGE INTESTINE Meridian (LI), SMALL INTESTINE Meridian (SI), BLADDER Meridian (BL), TRIPLE ENERGIZER Meridian (TE) and GALLBLADDER Meridian (GB) pass through this area. LARGE INTESTINE Meridian (LI) and TRIPLE ENERGIZER Meridian (TE) pass near the upper edge of the trapezius muscle, and SMALL INTESTINE Meridian (SI) passes covering the upper part of the scapula. Effect of treatment of TE$_5$ and TE$_8$ is regarded to connect with three YO-U$^{(Jp.)}$(YANG)$^{(Ch.)}$ meridians of upper extremities (LI, SI & TE).

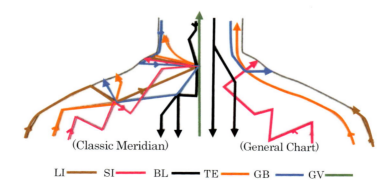

Fig.80-1 Meridians around "Shoulder"

Complaints around the upper edge of trapezius muscle, treatment of TE₂ or TE₃ is more effective. If the pain is around scapular region, it is better to add treatment of the point of SMALL INTESTINE Meridian (SI₃ etc.). For the pain around vertebra, treatment is the same as back of the neck

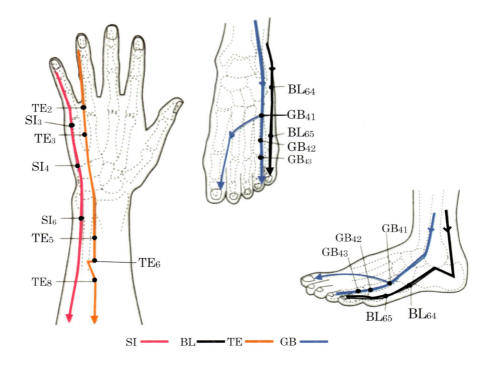

Fig.80-2 Points for Treatment of "Shoulder"

[2] Around the Shoulder Joint

LARGE INTESTINE Meridian (LI, on the joint), SMALL INTESTINE Meridian (SI)) & TRIPLE ENERGIZER Meridian (TE) (back of the joint) and LUNG Meridian (LU) & PERICARDIUM Meridian (PC) (anterior of the joint) pass around the shoulder joint.

Also by treatment of shoulder joint, it is very important to confirm the localization of the pain. It is to be remembered that locating the place of pain at the shoulder region is unexpectedly difficult.

In many cases, pain is complained on the shoulder joint around LI₁₅, but the pain at the anterior part of the shoulder joint is not rare. And pain at the anterior part of the joint is very often not realized by the patient. Pain of the shoulder joint is one of the most difficult places to confirm the exact localization of the pain. And, by not few cases, the place of pain changes in the course of treatment. So, by acupuncture treatment of this area, the localization of pain must be confirmed each time of treatment.

150 PART 6 PRACTICE OF ACUPUNCTURE

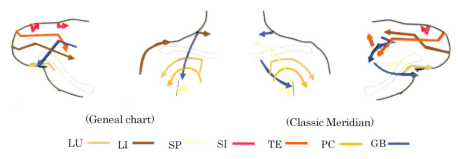

Fig.81-1 Meridians around Shoulder Joint

For the treatment of troubles around the shoulder joint, TE$_5$ or TE$_8$ which covers wide range of three Yo-u$^{(Jp.)}$ meridians (LI, SI, TE) is most convenient. When the localization of the pain is clear, it is better to add point of corresponding meridian. That is:

  Posterior part of shoulder joint: SI (SI$_3$, SI$_4$, SI$_6$ etc.)
  Anterior part of shoulder joint: LU (LU$_6$, LU$_7$ etc.)
As the customary of the treatment of every joint (mentioned later):
  KI (KI$_2$, KI$_7$ etc.)
  PC (PC$_5$, PC$_6$ etc.)
When the patient has pain on motion, there are other methods of treatment such as:
  Auricular acupuncture: Shoulder Joint to Shoulder
  Thumbtack Needle: At the points which the patient feels pain by motion.

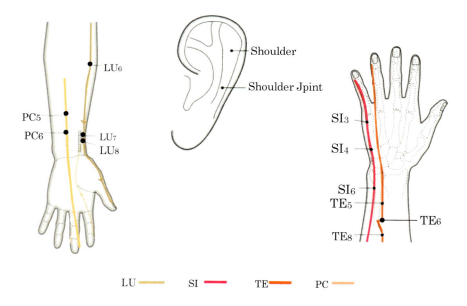

Fig.81-2 Points of Treatment for the Pain around Shoulder Joint

§ 6 Arm & Hand

[1] General Rule

Pathway of meridians of the upper extremity is simple, and their branches are very few. So, meridian selection is easy if the location of pain is clear. However, it should be noticed that the pathway of meridians, especially at forearm, changes markedly by pronation and supination as mentioned before (PART 3). Patients often indicate the place of pain by strongly pronated position, which leads the practitioner mistake the necessary meridian.

When the place of pain is wide or vague, or too many meridians are necessary for the treatment, "glaring all direction point" is very useful. For example, effects by the treatment of TE_5 or TE_8 is regarded to be transmitted to all YO-U$^{(Jp.)}$(YANG$^{(Ch.)}$) meridians (LI, SI and TE) and PC_5 and PC_6 to all IN$^{(Jp.)}$(YIN$^{(Ch.)}$) meridians (LU, HT and PC).

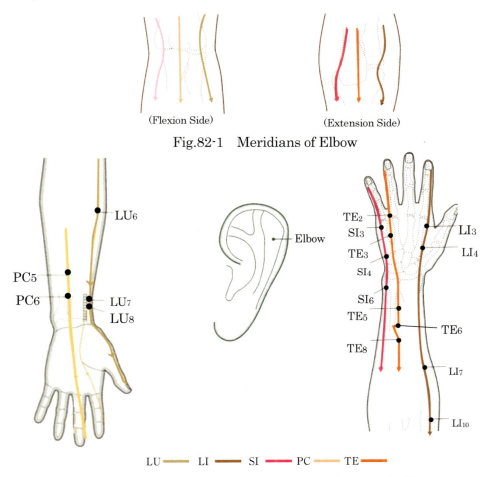

Fig.82-1　Meridians of Elbow

Fig.82-2　Meridians of Forearm & Hand and Points for Treatment

[2] Elbow Joint

Treatment of the pain of elbow joint is fairly difficult. Frequently used points are:

LARGE INTESTINE Meridian: LI$_4$, LI$_7$, LI$_{10}$
SMALL INTESTINE Meridian: SI$_3$, SI$_4$, (SI$_6$, mainly for acupoint injection)
TRIPLE ENERGIZER Meridian: TE$_3$, TE$_5$, TE$_8$
LUNG Meridian: LU$_6$, LU$_7$, LU$_8$
HEART Meridian: HT$_4$, HT$_5$
PERICARDIUM Meridian: PC$_5$, PC$_6$

If the effect is insufficient, auricular acupuncture is useful. Point to use is "Elbow". This point is fairly difficult to insert, and strict attention for disinfection is necessary.

Intradermal acupuncture or thumbtack needle is also useful. The method is the same as the shoulder joint pain. However, fixation of needle by intradermal acupuncture is difficult, and effect is somewhat uncertain. In most of cases, points of KIDNEY Meridian (KI$_2$ or KI$_7$) and PERICARDIUM Meridian (mostly PC$_5$) are also used together (mentioned later)

[3] Hand Joint & Fingers

Meridian & point selection is almost the same as the treatment of elbow joint. "Arm point" for hand joint and "Finger point" for finger in auricle are very difficult to use. The largest risk is that the needle penetrates till back of the auricle. So, by insertion, back of the auricle must be strictly disinfected before treatment.

§ 7   Anterior- & Lateral Chest

According to the classic literatures, all meridians except BLADDER Meridian and GOVERNOR VESSEL pass through this area. In general meridian charts, CONCEPTION VESSEL (CV), KIDNEY Meridian (KI), PERICARDIUM Meridian (PC), STOMACH Meridian (ST), SPLEEN Meridian (SP), GALLBLADDER Meridian (GB) and LIVER Meridian (LR) are illustrated here. Pathways of other meridians are not clear. They may pass deeper part of the body. Points for the treatment of this area are usually selected on the seven meridians of general meridian charts mentioned above.

Meridian- and point- selection is usually according to general rule, excluding exceptional cases as pain of coronary vascular event or intercostal neuralgia. Pain around sternum can be treated by points of KIDNEY Meridian (KI). Treatment of CONCEPTION VESSEL is almost needless. Treatment of STOMACH Meridian (ST) is effective for pain of the breast (mamma).

Frequently used points are as described below.
KIDNEY Meridian: KI$_2$, KI$_7$,
STOMACH Meridian: ST$_{36}$, ST$_{41}$, ST$_{43}$, ST$_{44}$
PERICARDIUM Meridian: PC$_5$, PC$_6$

SPLEEN Meridian: SP3, SP4, SP6, SP10
GALLBLADDER Meridian: GB35, GB41, GB42, GB43
LIVER Meridian: LR3, LR5, LR8

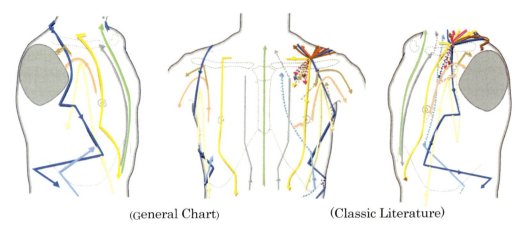

(General Chart)　　　　(Classic Literature)
Fig.83-1　Meridians of Anterior & Lateral Chest

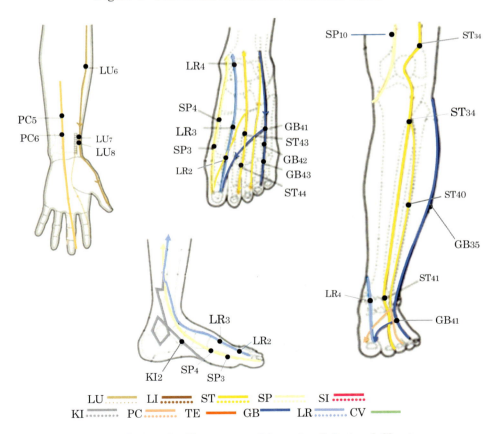

Fig.83-2　Points for Treatment of Anterior & Lateral Chest

154   PART 6   PRACTICE OF ACUPUNCTURE

§ 8   Abdominal Pain

In the treatment of abdominal pain, as mentioned before, diagnosis before treatment is most important. "Treatment without diagnosis" must be regarded as contraindication of acupuncture. Acupuncture therapy must be given after definite diagnosis or treatment for urgent severest pain. In this occasion, acupoint injection is more adequate than electro-acupuncture. Acupoint injection with strong analgesics or opiates can sedate severest pain. However, it must be noticed that acupuncture therapy can mislead diagnosis due to too strong analgesic effect.

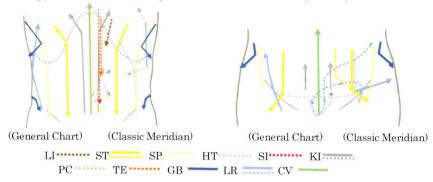

Fig.84-1   Meridian of abdomen & Inguinal Region

Meridian-and-point selection is always according to the general rule. Points for abdominal pain are shown in Fig.84-2.

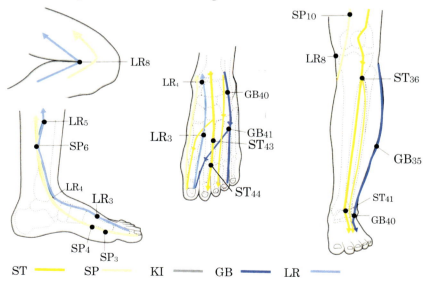

Fig.84-2   Points for Treatment of Abdomen & Inguinal Region

[1] Epigastrium (So Called "Stomachache")

In general meridian chart, CONCEPTION VESSEL (CV), KIDNEY Meridian (KI) and STOMACH Meridian (ST) are illustrated. According to the classic literatures, all meridians except BLADDER Meridian (BL) and GOVERNOR VESSEL (GV) pass here. Points of STOMACH Meridian (ST) and KIDNEY Meridian (KI) are mainly used with satisfactory effects. Sometimes points of SPLEEN Meridian (SP) and LIVER Meridian are used together (it is not so frequent).

Frequently used points are:
  STOMACH Meridian: ST_{36}, ST_{41}, ST_{43}, ST_{44}
  KIDNEY Meridian: KI_2, KI_7, (KI_3, KI_4, KI_5, KI_6 for acupoint injection)
  SPLEEN Meridian: SP_3, SP_4, SP_6, SP_{10}
  LIVER Meridian: LR_3, LR_8

[2] Hypochondrium

KIDNEY Meridian (KI), STOMACH Meridian (ST), SPLEEN Meridian (SP), GALLBLADDER Meridian (GB) and LIVER Meridian (LR) pass though this area. These pathways of general meridian chart, and classic literatures are not always the same.

Frequently used points are:
  KIDNEY Meridian: KI_2, KI_7, (KI_3, KI_4, KI_5, KI_6 for acupoint injection)
  STOMACH Meridian: ST_{36}, ST_{41}, ST_{43}, ST_{44}
  SPLEEN Meridian: SP_3, SP_4, SP_6, SP_{10} (Treatment of SP_6 or SP_{10}, often gives excellent effect with the treatment of one pair points.)
  GALLBLADDER Meridian: GB_{35}, GB_{41}, GB_{42}, GB_{43}
  LIVER Meridian: LR_3, LR_8

[3] Pain around Navel

In general meridian chart, CONCEPTION VESSEL (CV) and KIDNEY Meridian (KI) pass this area. According to the classic literatures, STOMACH Meridian (ST), SPLEEN Meridian (SP), TRIPLE ENERGIZER Meridian (TE) and PERICARDIUM Meridian (PC) pass here, but their pathways are not clear. The same method of acupuncture treatment of epigastrium (mentioned above) is effective.

[4] Lower Abdomen

In general meridian charts, CONCEPTION VESSEL (CV) KIDNEY Meridian (KI), STOMACH Meridian (ST), SPLEEN Meridian (SP), GALLBLADDER Meridian (GB) and LIVER Meridian (LR) are illustrated. About their pathways there are various opinions. Points for treatment in this area are the same points mentioned above ([1]~[3]).

[5] Inguinal Region (Fig.84)

In general meridian chart, STOMACH Meridian (ST), SPLEEN Meridian (SP) and LIVER Meridian (LR) pass through this area. According to the classic literatures, also GALLBLADDER Meridian (GB) passes here. For the treatment of lateral part, points of SPLEEN Meridian (usually SP_6 or SP_{10}), and for the median part, Stomach Meridian (ST_{36} or ST_{43} etc.) are used. At any part of this area, better effects are often obtained adding the points of LIVER Meridian (LR_3, LR_8 etc.).

§ 9 Back & Lumbar Pain

Pain of this region is one of the best indications of acupuncture.

Effect of electro-acupuncture is surest and long lasting, and acupoint injection is also very effective. Acupoint injection of pharmacologically inactive substances such as saline solution or vitamins often induces excellent and long lasting effect.

Acupuncture therapy for fresh injury is often difficult, because the patient hardly endure to keep same position for long a time, and the effect itself is not sure. However, for the compression fracture of vertebra, it is often useful. Probably because the patients with compression fracture of vertebra don't like moving and they can keep lying for a long time. So, treatment for a long time (often over one hour) is possible, and good effects are often obtained. For fresh injury, acupoint injection with analgesics (Pentazocine etc.) is more practical.

Meridians passing through this area are not so different between general meridian charts and classic literatures. Mainly GOVERNOR VESSEL (GV) & BLADDER Meridian (BL), and GALLBLADDER Meridian (GB) is concerned. In most cases, treatment of points of BLADDER Meridian (BL) produces excellent effect. Using points on GALLBLADDER Meridian (GB) together, better effects are expected. If the effect is insufficient, acupoint injection to GV_{14} is very effective.

Point selection of BLADDER Meridian has some tendency, though it is not absolute rule. That is: Proximal points (Bl_{58}, BL_{59}, BL_{60}) for the lumbar pain, and distal points (BL_{60} and Bl_{64} or BL_{65}) for the pain of the thoracic region.

For the pain around 3rd lumber vertebra, treatment of GB_{26} is very useful. But vertical insertion of this point is undesirable because of the risk to injure the abdominal viscera. So, treatment of this point is not easy for beginners except acupoint injection.

My method of point selection in this area is:

1) **Region of thoracic vertebra:**
   BL_{60}, BL_{64}
   & one of (GB_{41}, GB_{42} or GB_{43})
2) **Around 3rd lumber vertebra** (height of navel):
   BL_{59}, BL_{60} and GB_{26}
3) **Area from lower lumber vertebra to upper sacral region:**
   2 of BL_{58}, BL_{59} and BL_{60} + GB_{35}

Using electro-acupuncture, if GALLBLADDER Meridian (GB) is "excess" by pulse diagnosis, principally one point of GALLBLADDER Meridian (GB) is used independent from the position of the pain

Chapter 1 Pain (Including Stiffness & Numbness) 157

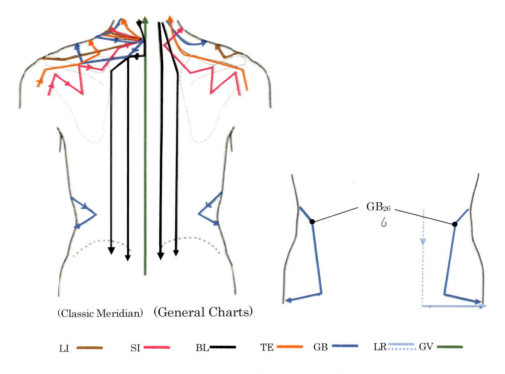

LI —— SI —— BL —— TE —— GB —— LR ····· GV ——

Fig 85-1 Meridians of Back- & Abdomen

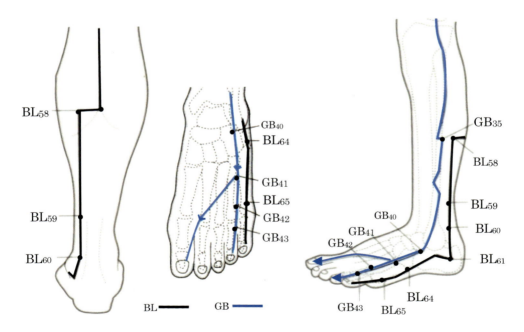

Fig.85-2 Points of Treatment for Back- & Lumber Region

§ 10 Sacral Region and around Gluteal Region

According to the classic literatures, GOVERNOR VESSEL (GV), BLADDER Meridian (BL) and GALLBLADDER Meridian (GB) pass here, and KIDNEY Meridian (KI) passes the tip of coccyx (GV_1). In general meridian charts, GALLBLADDER Meridian is described only in some meridian charts. Method of treatment is also the same as lower lumbar pain. When pain is around coccyx, a point of KIDNEY Meridian (KI_2 or KI_7) is added.

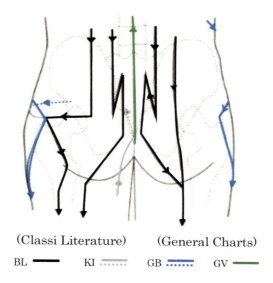

(Classi Literature)　(General Charts)
BL ───　KI ·····　GB ·····　GV ───

Fig.86　Meridians of Sacral- & Gluteal Region

§ 11　Genital Area and around Anus (Fig.87)

According to the classic literatures, GOVERNOR VESSEL (GV), KIDNEY Meridian (KI) and LIVER Meridian (LR) pass this area, and some classic literature says that CONCEPTION VESSEL passes here. LIVER Meridian (LR) is regarded to connect with genital organs. Their pathways in general meridian charts or dolls are fairly different, and in some charts, a pathway around the genital organ is absent.

In general charts, pathway of KIDNEY Meridian (KI) is not clear between median side of upper leg and KI_{11} (at the upper edge of pubic bone). Classic literatures say that KI-Meridian passes the tip of coccyx (GV_1), and "KIDNEY" has significant implication for reproductive function.

In these meanings, points of KIDNEY Meridian (KI_2 or KI_7) and LIVER Meridian (LR_3, LR_5 or LR_8) are used for the treatment of this area at first. As SP_6 and SP_{10} are regarded to have close connection with KI-Meridian and LR-Meridian, one of

Chapter 1 Pain (Including Stiffness & Numbness) 159

them is used with the treatment of this area. Symptoms of genital organ often disappear with the treatment of only SP6.

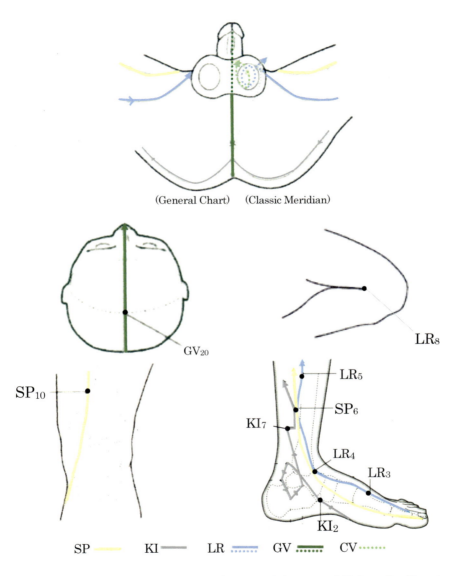

Fig.87 Meridians of Genital Area & around Anus and Points for Treatment

From ancient days, moxibustion to GV20 is used for the treatment of hemorrhoid. Acupuncture treatment of GV20 is effective, but as this part is covered with hair, disinfection is often difficult. For using GV20, acupoint injection is more convenient than electro-acupuncture.

160   PART 6   PRACTICE OF ACUPUNCTURE

§ 12   Lower Extremity

[1] Pain of the Leg

Pathways of meridians are fairly different among books and meridian charts. Especially pathways of BLADDER Meridian are not only between general meridian charts and classic literatures, but also between Japanese charts and Chinese meridian dolls (even between themselves) various differences are found. But according to any chart, good effects are obtained.

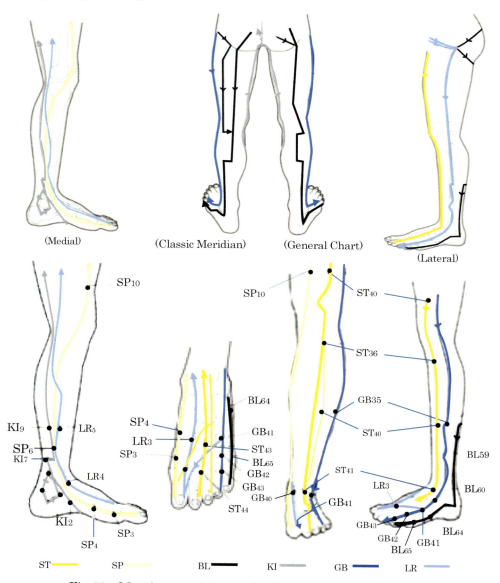

Fig.88   Meridians and Points for Treatment of Leg & Foot

1) Dorsal Side of the Leg

Pain in this area is often associated with lumbar pain, and almost same points for the treatments for lumbar pain are used also for the pain in this area. In my method, points of BLADDER Meridian (BL$_{58}$, BL$_{59}$ or BL$_{60}$) is mainly used, and secondarily points of GALLBLADDER Meridian (mainly GB$_{41}$ or GB$_{35}$) and KIDNEY Meridian (KI$_2$ or KI$_7$) are used.

2) Inner Side of the Leg

SPLEEN Meridian (SP), KIDNEY Meridian (KI) and LIVER Meridian (LR) pass through this area. SP$_6$ and SP$_{10}$ are regarded to connect with KI-Meridian and LR-Meridian, and treatment of only one of these two points often produces excellent effect. SP$_6$ or SP$_{10}$ is almost always used for the treatment in this area.

Otherwise, following points are often used.

KIDNEY Meridian: KI$_2$, KI$_7$

LIVER Meridian: LR$_3$, LR$_8$

3) Lateral Side of the Leg

GALLBLADDER Meridian (GB) passes center of this part, and STOMACH Meridian(ST) and BLADDER Meridian (BL) have some relationship with the complaints of this area. GB$_{35}$ is regarded to connect with ST-Meridian and BL-Meridian. And treatment of only GB$_{35}$ often produces good effect for the complaint in this area. GB$_{35}$ is almost always used for the treatment of this area. Otherwise, following points are often used too.

GALLBLADDER Meridian: GB$_{41}$, GB$_{42}$

STOMACH Meridian: ST$_{36}$, ST$_{43}$

BLADDER Meridian: BL$_{58}$, Bl$_{59}$, BL$_{60}$

4) When the Location of Pain is Too Wide or Indistinct

If all the meridians are deficient or excess, treatment of SP$_6$ and GB$_{35}$ are tried at first. Here acupoint injection is very useful. At first, vertical injection to SP$_6$ and GB$_{35}$ is tried using pharmacologically inactive substances such as saline solution or vitamin (B$_1$ or B$_{12}$). If the pain disappears, treatment of other points is not necessary. If pain remains, same injection is given to the points of other meridians one by one, and necessary meridians will become clear automatically. This is the easiest meridian selection.

[2] Pain in the Hip Joint (Fig.90)

GB$_{30}$ is the nearest point to the hip joint. According to the classic literature, GALLBLADDER Meridian (GB) and BLADDER Meridian (BL) pass here. Illustration of general meridian charts is various. Some describes only BL-Meridian, and someone describes GB- & BL- Meridians. Seeing from the front, SPLEEN Meridian (SP) passes near the head of the hip joint. From these points of view, points of BLADDER Meridian (BL$_{59}$ or BL$_{60}$) and GALLBLADDER Meridian (GB$_{35}$ or GB$_{41}$) are

162   PART 6   PRACTICE OF ACUPUNCTURE

used for the pain in the hip joint. According to the joint pain on motion, treatment of points on SPLEEN Meridian (SP$_6$ etc.) is added.

As mentioned later, for the treatment of joints, point on KIDNEY Meridian (KI$_2$, KI$_7$ etc.) and PERICARDIUM Meridian (PC$_5$ or PC$_6$) are principally used together.

When the treatment of body acupuncture is insufficient, treatment together with auricular needle (Hip Joint Point) is often effective, but it is not so often used.

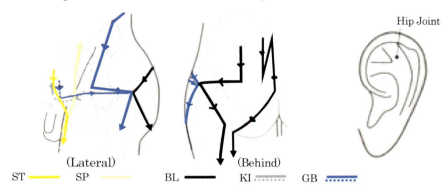

Fig.89   Meridians around Hip Joint and point of Auricle

[3] Pain in the Knee Joint

Pathways of meridian around the knee joint are almost the same in classic literatures and general meridian charts, and meridian selection according to the localization of the complaints is easy. However, the lesion of knee joint is often very broad unrelated to the symptom. So, for the treatment of the knee joint, it is better to treat overall part of the knee.

Basic point selection is SP$_6$, GB$_{35}$ and KI$_2$ or KI$_7$, and additionally, points of meridians that pass through the place of pain are treated. As the treatment for these additional points, moxa needle or acupoint injection is very useful. Although it is very rare, if effect of body acupuncture is insufficient, auricular acupuncture is useful. Points on the ear are "Knee" and "Knee Joint". Usually, short needle is inserted from "Knee" to "Knee Joint". Here attention must be strictly paid for disinfection.

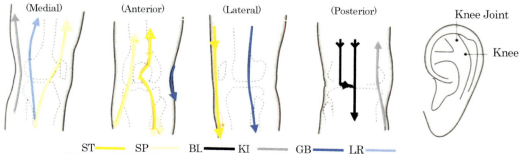

Fig.90   Meridians around Knee Joint and Points of the Auricle

[4] Pain of the Foot

Most of the pain of this area is neuralgia or arthritis. Pathways of meridians of this area are simple, and meridian selection due to the location of pain is easy. Combination of $SP_6 - GB_{35}$ is also useful here. For the pain in the joints, treatment of KI_2 or KI_7 and PC_5 or PC_6 are added. If the effect is insufficient, auricular acupuncture can be used. Point is "Foot Joint" and/or "Toe" or "Heel", according to the location of pain. But these points, especially "Toe" and "Heel", are very difficult to use.

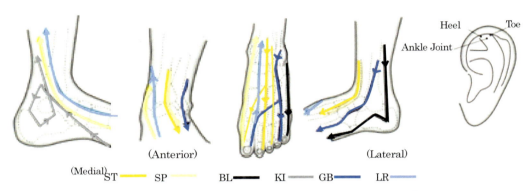

Fig.91 Meridians of Foot Joint and Points of Auricle

§ 13 Pain of Malignant Tumor

Pain due to malignant tumor is often very severe and persistent, and measures of its treatment are one of the important themes of the therapy of cancer.

Among the pain sedating methods, most commonly used method is analgesics, especially opiates. For the severest pain, intravenous drip infusion of large amount of opiates is performed. In my experience, cancer pain can be well sedated by acupoint injection with analgesics (especially opiates), together with mild cancer chemotherapy. In many cases, oral administration of opiates is difficult, and for severest pain, oral use of opiates is often not effective enough. Too much administration of morphine has many problems, and it is not desirable for the sake of patient's ADL.

Pain sedating effect of mild cancer chemotherapy is unexpectedly strong, and sometimes only with mild chemotherapy, pain can be considerably sedated. Not so strong pain can be sedated by mild analgesics as NSAIDs. Strong cancer chemotherapy is more effective. But it is difficult except specialists to use, and it is not so easy for patients in the end stage.

As mentioned before, acupuncture can sedate many kinds of pain. Cancer pain is not its exception. Meridian and point selection is very easy, only to choose meridians which pass through the place of the pain.

But there are some characteristic conditions as described below.

1) Electro-acupuncture is often difficult, and its effect is often insufficient.
2) Duration of the effect of acupuncture is short, at most a few days.
   (In my experience, when the duration of effect of acupuncture is unexpectedly short, the cause of the pain should be suspected diabetic pain or cancer.)
3) Acupoint injection is more useful than electro-acupuncture.

Acupoint Injection for Cancer Pain

My method of cancer pain sedation is to use analgesics (mainly opiates by acupoint injection) together with mild cancer chemotherapy. Acupoint injection for pain of malignant tumor has some characteristic conditions apart from the usual case as described below.

1) Frequent injection is necessary for long period.
   Frequent injection at the same point causes induration. So, attention is necessary not to use same point too frequently.
2) Analgesics, very often opiates, are necessary for injection.
3) Attention must be paid for sensory paralysis.

Method of Point Selection

Point selection is according to the principle that "To select points on the meridians that pass through the place of pain". However, it is not desirable "To select **always** same point" as mentioned before. Points of the same meridian have nearly the same character, and by acupoint injection of analgesics, the effect is not widely different.

As mentioned before, "acupuncture at anesthetic part" is ineffective, and injection at such point doesn't produce effect better than pharmacological effect. In such cases, treatment must be given at head or trunk. By acupoint injection, deep insertion is seldom necessary, but by injection at chest, risk of pneumothorax must be always kept in mind.

When the treatment is necessary for very long period, almost all points become indurated, and injection becomes difficult. In such case, "injection between two acupuncture points" sometimes produces excellent effect showing marked phenomenon of "flow".

Medicaments for Injection

Strength of analgesia is different medication by medication. For acupoint injection for cancer pain, pharmacologically effective medication is necessary. For severe pain, stronger opiates must be used, but for not so severe pain, non-narcotic analgesics such as Pentazocine are often enough effective.

Effect of Acupoint Injection

Effect appears promptly, usually within several seconds. Using strong opiates, whatever severe pain can be sedated immediately, and its effect continues at least about 8 hours. I have no experience of case that I had to give injection of opiates over 4 times a day.

There is no need to worry about addiction. Even a patient who got 387 ampules (1ml/ampule) of opiate for one year and a half, addiction did not appear at all.

Chapter 2 Acupuncture in Surgery, Orthopedics & Anesthesiology

In this chapter, pain &/or stiffness or numbness is most frequently appear as the symptom, and the methods of acupuncture treatment overlap with what is mentioned in Chapter 1. If the description of this chapter is unsatisfactory, please refer to the description of Chapter 1.

§ 1 Acupuncture Related to Operation

[1] Acupuncture as Premedication

Premedication has many purposes. For the purpose to elevate the threshold of pain, acupoint injection is very useful. For premedication, usually opiates or Pentazocine is used. Using these medications in the form of acupoint injection, pain-sedating effect is remarkably strengthened and its duration is remarkably extended. Meridian & point selection for acupoint injection is the same as mentioned in Part 1, supposing the pain is around operating field. It is quite easy.

I have an experience of hysterectomy for a patient with uterine myoma who cannot receive Halothane due to the liver disease. Outline was as described below.

Inhalation anesthetic: $NO_2 + O_2$

Used medication: Pethidine Hydrochloride (35mg, 1ml ampule)

Point selection: SP_6, ST_{36}, FKI_7

Effect: Reflex for pain disappeared rapidly, and the course of anesthesia was very smooth. As the muscle relaxant drug, only SCC (Succinyl Choline Chloride) was used, and its total dose was remarkably less than by usual laparotomy using halothane.

[2] Acupuncture for Postoperative Pain

Recently continuous epidural anesthesia is often used for sedation of postoperative pain. But injection of analgesics or opiates is also often used. If the injection is given in the form of acupoint injection, long lasting effect appears rapidly with smaller dose. Point selection is easily determined according to the location of pain as mentioned in Part 1. For this purpose, acupoint injection is much better than electro-acupuncture.

[3] Acupuncture for Postoperative Paresis of Intestine

Prolonged wind due to intestinal paresis after the laparotomy often causes patient's distress. Marked accelerating effect of dispersing wind is often given by acupoint injection of Vitamin B_1 or V. B_{12}. Points are LI_4, LI_7 or LI_{10} (including pleural use). Treatment of LI_{10} is very effective. But this point deviates markedly by pronation, and it is not always easy to find this point for beginners.

166　PART 6 PRACTICE OF ACUPUNCTURE

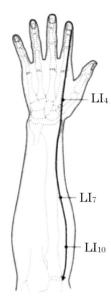

Fig.92　Points for treatment of Intestinal Paresis

[4] Acupuncture Anesthesia

Acupuncture anesthesia was developed during The Great Cultural Revolution in China. It is difficult to get literatures of acupuncture anesthesia. Fortunately, I had one chance to observe it in China. It seemed to be combination of body acupuncture and local acupuncture under strong premedication.

The difference between usual acupuncture therapy and acupuncture anesthesia is as described below.

1) Thick and long needle over No.34 (0.34mm in diameter) is used regardless of deficiency or excess.
2) In addition to usual pain sedating points, two dick long needles are inserted parallel to incision line for electric stimulation.
3) Stimulation with 3 Hz rectangular (spike?) wave as strong as the patient can endure.
4) As premedication, relatively large dose of analgesics as Pentazocine or opiates is used.
5) Method is only electric acupuncture.

They say that acupuncture anesthesia has many merits. The greatest demerits are uncertainty of effect and inefficiency. At least in my experience, although the threshold of pain evidently elevated, "complete painless" is hardly obtained without very strong premedication, and it takes time so much. From the beginning of start of stimulation to the beginning of surgical operation, it takes at least 30 minutes.

§ 2 Acupuncture Therapy for Fresh Injury

[1] General Fresh Injury (Wound, Fracture etc.)

Effect of electro-acupuncture for the fresh injury is not so evident. If suitable stimulation is given continuously for long time as acupuncture anesthesia, some effect may be obtained. But it is not practical.

Expected effect of acupuncture for the fresh injury may be obtained by acupoint injection. For this purpose, saline solution or vitamin is not effective enough, and usually strong analgesics as Pentazocine is necessary.

[2] Compression Fracture of Vertebra

Usually analgesic effect of acupuncture is weak for fresh fracture. But for the compression fracture of vertebra, acupuncture is fairly effective. As patients of vertebral fracture like to keep spine position immobile, long time treatment of electro-acupuncture can be easily given. Using electric stimulation over 30 minutes (over one hour, if possible) to Bl_{60}, BL_{64} & GB_{41} and moxa needle for KI_2, good effect is obtained

Acupoint injection with strong analgesics as Pentazocine is also effective. Sometimes immediate walking is possible just after the injection. Pleural points of BLADDER Meridian (BL_{59}, BL_{60}, BL_{64}, BL_{65} etc.) and GALLBLADDER Meridian (GB_{35}, GB_{41}, GB_{42} etc.) are selected.

As most of the patients of this fracture have osteoporosis, usually point of KIDNEY Meridian (KI_2, KI_7 etc.) is treated together. GV_{14} is difficult to use for electro-acupuncture.

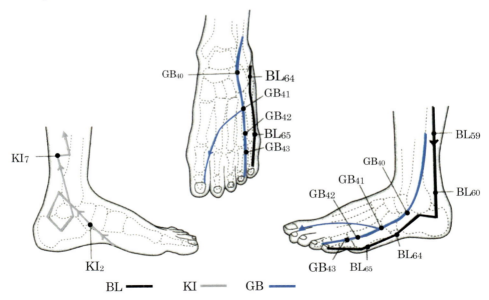

Fig.93 Points for Treatment of Vertebral Compression Fracture

§ 3　Refractory Fistula

Fistulas sometimes become intractable, and, for the radical cure, large scale surgical operation is necessary. I have experiences of refractory fistula after surgical operation of peritonitis (due to appendicitis) and anal fistula. They were successfully cured by acupuncture except one case of anal fistula. In this exceptional case, although complete cure was not achieved, the fistula was found to be unexpectedly good state at the radical operation.

Method of treatment is electro-acupuncture, and point selection is the points on the meridians that pass through the part of the fistula. Stimulation is supplementation or draining according to deficiency or excess of the meridians, and frequency of the treatment is two or three times a week.

§ 4　Whiplash Syndrome

The most frequently complained symptom of the whiplash syndrome is pain and stiffness of the neck and the shoulder. Furthermore many symptoms such as headache or dull headache, pain &/or numbness of the arm, lumber or back pain, nausea, dizziness, tinnitus, pain of the eye, photophobia, lacrimation, impotence or general fatigue and so on. Almost all of these symptoms, except general fatigue, are easily treated by acupuncture. Whiplash syndrome is one of the best indications of acupuncture.

[1] Method of Treatment

The first choice of treatment is electro-acupuncture.

Almost all cases of whiplash syndrome have stiffness &/or pain of the neck and the shoulder as chief complaint. Stiffness of shoulder is mainly complained around the upper edge of the trapezius, but it is often claimed also on the scapular- or inter-scapular region. BLADDER Meridian (BL), TRIPLE ENERGIZER Meridian (TE) and GALLBLADDER Meridian (GB) pass through this area. So, the fundamental meridian selection is these three meridians. For the other symptoms, points of each suitable meridian are treated, by way of moxa needle etc.

Point selections are as described below.

1) Fundamental Points (For stiffness of neck &/or shoulder)

BLADDER Meridian; BL_{64}

TRIPLE ENERGIZER Meridian: TE_5 (or TE_8)

GALLBLADDER Meridian: GB_{41} or GB_{43}

2) Back- or Lumber- Pain or Headache

Points for treatment are almost the same as the fundamental condition. If lumbar pain is very strong, BL_{59} or BL_{60} is used for electric stimulation and BL_{64} is treated by moxa needle.

3) Tinnitus &/or Dizziness

Point selection for tinnitus &/or dizziness is as following order.

Fundamental points + TE$_5$ or TE$_8$ → + TE$_2$ or TE$_3$ → + GB$_{41}$ or GB$_{43}$

If the effect is insufficient, moxa needle of KI$_2$ is added. Auricular acupuncture (Inner Ear Point) may be effective, but I have no chance to use it.

4) Symptoms of the Eye (Pain, Photophobia, Lacrimation, Diplopia etc.)

Fundamental points + LR$_3$ Sometimes CV22, HT5, auricular point (Eye Point) are added by acupoint injection.

5) Nausea

Fundamental points + SP$_4$

6) Impotence

Treatment of SP$_6$ is often effective. Adding points of KIDNEY Meridian (KI$_2$ etc.) and LIVER Meridian (LR$_3$ etc.), effect is strengthened. Usually acupuncture treatment of impotence is difficult, but impotence by whiplash syndrome is relatively effective.

7) General Fatigue

Treatment of ST$_{36}$ and SP$_6$ is effective to some degree, but it is better to use Kampo$^{(Jp.)}$ medicine together.

Symptoms of whiplash syndrome are often various, and deficiency and excess of meridians are often complicated. If the symptoms are too many so as it is difficult to treat all of them at one time, the best way is to treat fundamental points and one or two other complaints. To treat other symptoms, treatment with acupoint injection is recommended. But as acupoint injection is fairly painful, it has a risk that the patient may come to dislike acupuncture.

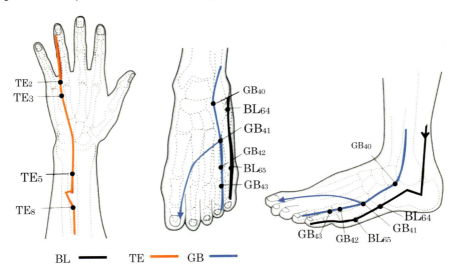

Fig.94 Fundamental Points for Treatment of Whiplash Injury

[2] Effect and Process of Acupuncture Therapy

Effect of acupuncture for whiplash syndrome usually appears rapidly. Almost all patients feel remarkable improvement during or just after the treatment. Sometimes the patient feels as if completely cured. But, soon after the treatment, complaints appear again. Some patient feels that complaints became worse due to the comparison phenomenon for the best state.

By the next treatment, complaints lessen or disappear immediately, and the effect diminishes gradually. Usually, the grade of recurrent complaint is less than by the previous treatment. And the time of duration of the effect becomes longer with every treatment. This process must be well explained before the start of the treatment.

The relation between the effect and frequency of treatment is evident. Between the effect of the treatment of "one time over a week" and "once a week" is decisive. Between "once a week" and "twice a week" is evident, and between "twice a week" and "thrice a week" difference is sometimes remarkable, but not always. So, it is recommended to receive acupuncture at least twice a week. Of course the effect of acupuncture is the more frequently the better.

State of visiting clinic has some tendency (Fig. 95).
1) For the beginning, patients visit clinic regularly as directed.
2) After a few weeks, visiting becomes gradually irregular.
    The reason of delay is usually "because of busy" or "because of inconvenience", and scarcely "because of improvement".
3) After several weeks, visiting becomes extremely irregular.
    When the patient visits clinic, the reason is usually "recurrence of symptoms due to weather or overwork".
4) The patient stops visiting while the practitioner is unaware. When the present state of the patient is clear, the patient is recovered completely.

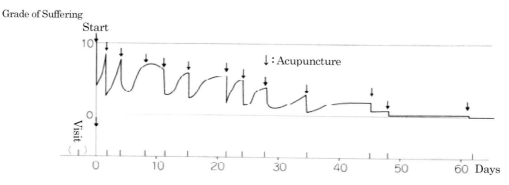

Fig.95 Typical Course of Visiting Clinic

Relation between the start of treatment and the effect is evident. That is: "The earlier the better". The effects of later started patients, especially over one month, are evidently inferior to the earlier started patients.

Effect for Barre Liu Syndrome is inferior.

[3] **Acupoint Injection for Whiplash Syndrome**

Acupoint injection is also effective for whiplash syndrome. Any substances can be used successfully. Usually analgesic medicament is not necessary, and Vitamin B_{12} is mainly used. However, as acupoint injection is fairly painful, and the therapy often takes long period, it is better to use acupoint injection only as supportive use.

§ 5 Cervicobrachial Syndrome & Thoracic Outlet Syndrome

Main symptom is stiffness of shoulder &/or numbness of the arm etc. like whiplash syndrome. And the same treatment is always effective. However, complaints of these diseases are caused by morphological change of bone or vertebra. So, duration of effect is usually short, and permanent cure by acupuncture is hardly expected. Attention should be paid if further treatment by Occidental Medicine is necessary.

§ 6 Lumber & Back Pain (cf. p157)

Acupuncture is very effective for lumber and back pain as mentioned before.

Many diseases cause lumber pain or back pain, and the diagnosis is not always easy. The method of acupuncture treatment is determined by the symptom, indifferent from the original disease. So, the method of acupuncture therapy is very easy, and it can be applied without diagnosis. But there are many diseases of lumber or back pain which must be treated by Occidental Medicine. It may be not unreasonable to treat such patient with acupuncture for pain sedation. But attention should be paid not to delay diagnosis.

Main meridians for the treatment of this pain are BLADDER Meridian (BL) and GALLBLADDER Meridian (GB) as mentioned in Chapter 1. If the patient has osteoporosis, KIDNEY Meridian (KI_2, KI_7 etc.) is treated together. For the coexisting neuralgia, corresponding meridians are treated together.

My standard of point selection is as mentioned below. But it is not a definite rule.

1) Pain at Lower Lumber Vertebra to Sacral Region:
    Electric Stimulation: BL_{58}, BL_{59}, GB_{35}
2) Pain around Coccygeal Bone
    Electric Stimulation: BL_{59}, GB_{35}, KI_2
3) Pain around 3rd Lumber Vertebra (Height of the navel)
    Electric Stimulation: BL_{58}, BL_{59}, GB_{26}

4) Pain at Thoracic Vertebra:
   Electric Stimulation: BL_{60}, BL_{64}, GB_{41}
(Moxa Needle for KI_2 is almost always used together.)
Acupoint injection to GV_{14} alone is often very effective.

§ 7   Spinal Canal Stenosis

Main symptoms of spinal canal stenosis are lumbar pain, neuralgia of the leg and intermittent claudication. Acupuncture treatment is as mentioned in preceding section and next Chapter. Electro-acupuncture for BL_{58}, BL_{59} & GB_{35} and Moxa Needle for KI_2 is usually used with good effect. Deformity of spinal canal cannot be cured by acupuncture. But, in many cases, while continuing treatment, the symptoms are relieved gradually, sometimes completely.

§ 8   Acupuncture Therapy for Articular Pain

One of the urgent desires of patients suffering from articular diseases is "relief from pain and motor disturbance". Treatment of these complaints is also important therapy, and here acupuncture is a reliable method of treatment.

The principle of the treatment is the same as mentioned in PART 1. Practical point selection for each joint is mentioned before. The most important condition is to confirm the location of the pain. Especially at shoulder joint, effect of misjudge of the location is evident.

There are many kinds of articular diseases. Recently, methods of treatment in Occidental Medicine have achieved marked development. They are different according to each disease, and many methods of operation have been put into practice. It may be reckless to attempt to cure all articular diseases with acupuncture.

If effect of body acupuncture is insufficient, auricular acupuncture is often useful. Points and insertion of auricular acupuncture are as described below.

   Shoulder joint: "Shoulder Joint" to "Shoulder"
   Elbow joint: "Elbow" to "Arm (may be meant hand joint)"
   Hand joint: "Arm joint" (In some chart it is written "Arm")
   Hip joint: "Hip joint"
   Knee joint: "Knee" to "Knee joint"
   Foot joint: "Ankle joint" to "Heel"

Chapter 2 Acupuncture in Surgery, Orthopedics & Anesthesiology   173

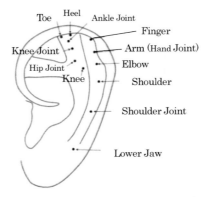

Fig.96   Points of Auricle for Treatment of Joints

There are points of phalangeal joints (hand and foot). But these points are at the top of the auricle. They are very difficult to insert, and aseptic manipulation is also difficult.

For the treatment of articular diseases, steroid hormones are often used with good effects. As mentioned before, KIDNEY may not be kidney but it closely resembles adrenal body. So, by the acupuncture treatment of articular diseases, principally point of KIDNEY Meridian (KI$_2$ or KI$_7$) is used together with usual body acupuncture. (This will be mentioned again in Chapter 12.)

For the treatment of the articular diseases, thumbtack needle is often useful. Meridian and point selection is the same as electro-acupuncture. Another method of thumbtack needle is only to put needle at the point where the patient feels pain by movement of the joint. This method is sometimes very effective.

Chapter 3 Diseases of Nervous System

§ 1 Central Nervous System

Acupuncture therapy is useful for the treatment of cerebrovascular disease, for the pain or the motor paralysis as mentioned before. Recently the mechanism of some diseases is clarified as autoimmune disease, and some of them are expected to be good target of acupuncture. They will be explained later.

Injury of the central nervous system often causes obstinate pain such as thalamic pain etc. It is very difficult to cure with my method of acupuncture.

§ 2 Neuralgia

Many kinds of disorders due to injury are successfully treated by acupuncture as mentioned before. Here, so called "Neuralgia" will be concerned.

Most of "neuralgia" is not the name of disease but the name of a symptom, and the right way of therapy is to cure the original disease. However, "to cure the pain" has also great clinical meaning, and acupuncture is very useful in this point. Method is only to treat the points on the meridians that pass through the place of the pain, regardless of the original disease. There is no risk of misdiagnose nor technical problem.

[1] **Trigeminal Neuralgia and Diseases with Similar Symptom**

There are many diseases that have pain at the region of trigeminal nerve, besides idiopathic trigeminal neuralgia. Methods of treatment in Occidental medicine are different according to the original disease. But their differential diagnosis is often very difficult, and misdiagnosis can causes grave consequence.

Recently therapeutic method of trigeminal neuralgia, such as Gasser's ganglion block or operation, has been developed markedly, and the effect is marvelous. However, its major premise is exact diagnosis, and the technique of the treatment is very difficult. Diagnosis seems not so difficult so long as the diagnosis is performed according to the diagnostic manual, but existence of confusing case cannot be denied. From such point of view, treatment of trigeminal neuralgia seems impossible except restricted specialists. However, there are many cases who want only relief from the pain. For such cases, acupuncture is very useful.

"For the complaints from different causes, same method based on the same principle is possible," is outstanding merit of acupuncture. The method of acupuncture therapy of trigeminal neuralgia is only to treat the points of the meridian that passes through the place of the pain. Here, so far as the judgment of the location of the pain is clear, meridian selection is easy. Usually electro-acupuncture is used, and acupoint injection of Vitamin B_{12} is also effective.

Relation between localization of the pain and point selection is as described below:

Area of the 1st branch (NV$_I$)
GALLBLADDER Meridian: One of GB$_{41}$ or GB$_{42}$ or GB$_{43}$
TRIPLE ENERGIZEr Meridian: TE$_2$ or TE$_3$
BLADDER Meridian: BL$_{64}$ or BL$_{65}$

Area of the 2nd branch (NV$_{II}$)
STOMACH Meridian: ST$_{43}$ or ST$_{44}$
SMALL INTESTINE Meridian: SI$_3$ or SI$_4$
GALLBLADDER Meridian: One of GB$_{41}$, GB$_{42}$ or GB$_{43}$

Besides 3 meridians mentioned above, sometimes point of TRIPLE ENERGIZER Meridian (TE$_3$ or TE$_5$) is used, mainly by moxa needle.

Sometimes, one treatment of moxa needle at ST$_7$ of opposite side shows marvelous effect. It is worth while trying it, if the patient is not anxious about bleeding.

Area of the 3rd branch (NV$_{III}$)
STOMACH Meridian: ST$_{43}$ or ST$_{44}$
LARGE INTESTINE Meridian: LI$_4$ etc.
Ear: Lower Joe

Effect of acupuncture for the pain at the region of trigeminal nerve is always good. Often it is inferior to the effect of successfully performed Gasser's ganglion block, but fairly severe pain can be sedated by acupuncture immediately, and usually the effect continues for at least several days. Sometimes the pain disappears completely by one acupuncture treatment. When the pain relapses, each time the same method of acupuncture is given with good effect. Acupuncture is quite harmless except the insertion pain. It may be the best merit of acupuncture.

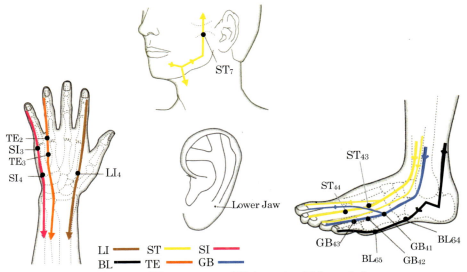

Fig.97 Points of Treatment of Trigeminal Neuralgia

It is very important not to overlook cancer pain. Duration of the effect for the cancer pain is fairly short. Usually it continues at most for a few days. But I have one experience of exception that the effect continued for one week for a patient of maxillary cancer. By the treatment of pain of this area, the existence of malignant tumor must be always kept in mind.

[2] Intercostal Neuralgia

Cause of the intercostal neuralgia is often at the thoracic vertebra, and in many cases, therapy of Occidental Medicine should be prioritized. In acupuncture treatment, attention should be paid not to overlook such lesions. However, acupuncture is enough useful and meaningful for the purpose of pain sedation.

The principle of treatment is to treat points on the meridians that pass through the place of pain as described below:

Back: BLADDER Meridian (BL) (often + GALLBLADDER Meridian (GB))
Lateral Chest: GALLBLADDER meridian (GB) and SPLEEN Meridian (SP)
Anterior Chest: KIDNEY Meridian (KI), SPLEEN Meridian (SP),
       LIVER Meridian (LR), GALLBLADDER Meridian (GB)

In the intercostal neuralgia, usually pain expands to the region of pleural meridians. So, it is often difficult to treat all meridians with electro-acupuncture. When the pain is spread in broad area, most convenient method is to use "glaring all directions point" as SP_6 or GB_{35}, and remaining complaints are treated stimulating points of suitable meridians with moxa needle or acupoint injection. Regardless of the location of neuralgic pain, adding treatment of point of BLADDER Meridian (BL_{64} or BL_{65}), often better effect is obtained.

Frequently used points for intercostal neuralgia are:

STOMACH Meridian: ST_{36}, ST_{43}, ST_{44}
SPLEEN Meridian: SP_3, SP_4, SP_6, SP_{10}
BLADDER Meridian: BL_{64}, BL_{65}
KIDNEY Meridian: KI_2, KI_7
GALLBLADDER Meridian: GB_{41}, GB_{42}, GB_{43}
LIVER Meridian: LR_3, LR_5

[3] Sciatica

The majority of sciatica originates in the lesion of lumbar vertebra, and very often it appears with lumbar pain. Acupuncture treatment of sciatica is almost the same as treatment of the lumbar pain (p.156). Location of pain of sciatica is mostly at the back &/or lateral side of the leg, but sometimes it is complained at the inner side. In this case, adding treatment of SP_6 better effect is obtained.

[4] Post-herpetic Neuralgia (PHN)

Herpes Zoster often causes severest pain. This pain disappears spontaneously in some patients, but very often the pain remains for a long time after the exanthema completely disappeared. This remained pain is called "post-herpetic neuralgia

(PHN)", and it is often very severe. This pain is often regarded to be incurable, but it can be relieved by acupuncture considerably.

The definition of PHN is mainly regarded as "the pain remained over 3months after the onset of Herpes Zoster". But, the effect of acupuncture differs according to the starting time of acupuncture therapy. In one word, it is "the sooner the better". By the patients who started acupuncture after more than one month from the onset of disease, the effect is evidently inferior to the patients who started treatment within one month. (Table6). So, the patients who have neuralgia after one month from the onset of Herpes Zoster may be better to be regarded as PHN.

Table 6 Relation between Effect and Onset of Disease (O) to Acupuncture (A)

(Including drop-out patients)

Time from O to A	<2 weeks	<1 month	<3months
Excellent Effect	104/114(91.2%)	26/40(65%)	11/32(34%)
>Good Effect	108/114(94.7%)	34/40(85%)	20/32(62.5%)
Time from O to A	<6 months	<1 year	>1 year
Excellent Effect	4/11(36.4%)	2/6(33.3%)	7/20(35%)
>Good Effect	7/11(63.6%)	2/6(33.3%)	14/20(70%)

Principle of the treatment is the same as the basic principle of the treatment of pain, namely it is to treat points on the meridians that pass thorough the location of the pain. Meridian selection is usually very easy. Method of treatment is mostly electro-acupuncture. Acupoint injection is also effective. However, as the treatment of PHN must be frequently, and it takes often very long time, and acupoint injection is fairly painful, it is rather difficult.

Progress of effect of treatment for PHN has special characteristics:

1) **Subsequent effect is often poor.**

Subsequent effect of acupuncture for fresh Herpes Zoster is remarkable without exception. But many patients of PHN do not feel any improvement just after the treatment. Patient of fresh Herpes Zoster realizes the effect the severer the pain the more vividly. But many patients of PHN are not aware of the subsequent effect of acupuncture, and the severer the pain the less the patient feels the effect.

2) **Rebound phenomenon seldom appears.**

Patients of fresh Herpes Zoster feel rebound phenomenon after the treatment almost without exception (mentioned later). But by PHN, evident rebound phenomenon seldom appears as if the treatment is effective.

3) Subjective improvement is poor as if objective improvement is evident.

Pain scale can be rated only by the patients themselves. However, the grade of the improvement is often better evaluated objective. Patients with PHN have an aversion to touch the painful part, and the patient moves slowly so as not to be rubbed by clothes. As the pain becomes milder, the patient moves more actively, and improvement of the patient is recognized by third people. But, at this period, the patient feels "not improved at all". And the patient becomes upset for the word "improved", answering "pain can be evaluated only by myself!". When the patient feels "a little bit improved", it can be evaluated as markedly improved.

4) "Frequent and Regular Treatment for Long Time" is necessary.

The most important condition of successful treatment for PHN is to continue treatment regularly until the pain disappears completely, at least the pain is relieved markedly so as the patient feels tolerable. When the patient cannot realize the effect, continuous treatment is very hard.

There are four cases of long time treatment of severe PHN. Comparing these cases, some specific feature is observed.

Case1. 85y.o. female

This case was treated by visiting treatment. Regular treatment is very difficult, and sometimes interval of treatment was over 3 weeks. Finally the treatment was ineffective in spite of the treatment for 7 years and a half.

Case2. 67y.o. male

This case was given focused treatment for about 2 weeks intermittently. Interval of each course was about 1 month. At the end of the course, the patient felt some effect, but at the next visit, pain was almost the same as before previous treatment. Finally the treatment was ineffective

Case3. 59y.o. female (Start of treatment: 2y.7m. after the onset of the disease)

This is the severest case in my experience. She was admitted to psychiatric hospital because of the incomprehensive pain. Electro-acupuncture therapy was given frequently, often every day, at least 3 times a week. After about one year, her pain became a little bit less serious. Thereafter her pain lessened gradually up to the grade "enough tolerable" after half a year of her "slightest improvement".

Case4. 77y.o. female (Start of treatment: 2 weeks after the onset of the disease)

At the period of this case, acupuncture treatment could perform only once a week, and we did not aware of the importance of frequent treatment for Herpes Zoster. So, PHN could not be prevented in spite of early start of the treatment. But fortunately PHN was completely cured with regular treatment for long-term (3years and 5months) under a good cooperation of the patient.

From these experiences we learned a lesson about the treatment of PHN.

It is **to continue treatment**

1. As frequently as possible,   2. Without interrupting treatment,
3. Regularly,   4. Until satisfactory effect is obtained.

After recovery from pain, slight relapse and fluctuation of pain appear in some patients. But severe pain never reappears. There is no case of recurrence of pain among completely (at least almost completely) cured patients.

This phenomenon has an important meaning from the viewpoint of treatment of PHN. Namely, many patients have to endure frequent and regular acupuncture therapy for a long time, bearing physical and economical pain, and feeling that the treatment is ineffective at all. Without enough comprehension of the patient and the family on this phenomenon, it is very difficult to complete the PHN therapy. Most of failure cases are dropout owing to the lack of comprehension about this condition.

[5] Diabetic Neuralgia

Principle of treatment is the same as the treatment of other neuralgia, and its effects are always excellent. But duration of the effect is usually very short. The effect scarcely continues more than two days. There are very few cases of long time treatment with fairly good effect. It looks like the process of post-herpetic neuralgia (PHN). Regular treatment for long time may be effective.

§ 3 Motor Paralysis

Cause of motor paralysis is often evident, and the method of treatment by Occidental Medicine is established in many cases. These cases should be treated by Occidental Medicine. However, there are some cases in whom the cause is not clear or the effect of treatment by Occidental Medicine is not enough effective. For such cases, acupuncture is often useful. Here, acupuncture therapy for the paralysis of skeletal muscle will be mentioned.

For the "apparent paralysis due to pain", acupuncture is very effective and useful. Method is the same as the treatment of pain as mentioned before.

The principle of the treatment for "real paralysis" is to select points on the meridians that pass through the location of paralyzed muscles and nerves that predominate the paralyzed muscle. Body acupuncture combined with eyelid acupuncture (p.120) is sometimes very effective.

Paralysis of the motor nerves is often accompanied with sensory paralysis. It is common sense that acupuncture is ineffective at the sensory paralyzed part. So, in such case, point must be selected at the sensory intact place. The method of treatment is usually electro-acupuncture, but acupoint injection of Vitamin B_{12} is sometimes effective.

[1] Facial Nerve Paralysis (Fig.98)

Many methods of treatment are performed for facial paralysis by Occidental Medicine such as application of vitamins or steroid hormones, physical therapy or stellate ganglion block etc. are performed with excellent effects. Among facial nerve paralysis, Bell's palsy is a benign disease and often spontaneously recovers. But most of patients who want acupuncture treatment are those who cannot get satisfactory effect by Occidental Medicine. Acupuncture therapy is often effective for such cases, and acupuncture has almost no side effects.

Treatment of Ramsey-Hunt Syndrome is often regarded to be very difficult, but excellent effect can be widely expected by acupuncture, especially for fresh cases. Often it is cured only by acupuncture. Prognosis of the traumatic paralysis is usually not so good. But in some cases, unexpected effect is obtained by acupuncture. Both types may be regarded as good indication of acupuncture. I have no experience of facial nerve paralysis due to injury of central nervous system.

Method of treatment is always the same independent of the cause of paralysis. There are three methods of point selection, namely direct stimulation to facial nerve, auricular acupuncture and body acupuncture (stimulation of suitable points of extremities)

In the face, vascular formation is abundant, and puncture of the face has a risk of bleeding and bruise formation. So, mainly body acupuncture is used, sometimes together with auricular acupuncture.

Meridian & point selection at extremities are:
- STOMACH Meridian: ST_{43}, ST_{44}
- SMALL INTESTINE Meridian: SI_3, SI_4
- TRIPLE ENERGIZER Meridian: TE_2, TE_3
- GALLBLADDER Meridian: GB_{41}, GB_{42}, GB_{43}
- LIVER Meridian: LR_3

When the treatment of extremities is not enough effective, points at face are exceptionally used under patient's enough comprehension as described below:
- STOMACH Meridian: ST_7
- SMALL INTESTINE Meridian: SI_{19}
- TRIPLE ENERGIZER Meridian: TE_{21}
- GALLBLADDER Meridian: GB_2
- Point of Auricle: Area of Face & Cheek

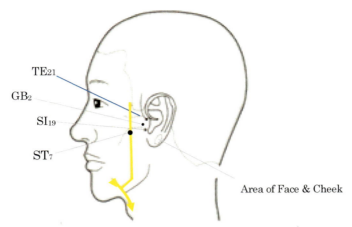

Fig.98-1   Points for Treatment of Facial Nerve Paralysis (Face & Ear)

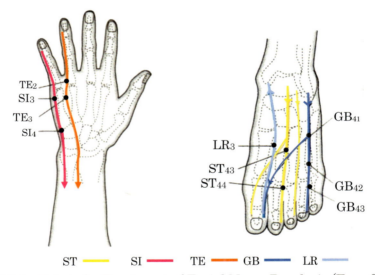

Fig.98-2   Points for Treatment of Facial Nerve Paralysis (Face & Foot)

[2] Recurrent Nerve Paralysis

Main complaint of recurrent nerve paralysis is hoarseness. When hoarseness is improved, almost all the aim has been achieved, at least for the patient. Acupuncture is often unexpectedly effective for hoarseness caused by recurrent nerve paralysis. For this purpose, usually electro-acupuncture is used, but acupoint injection of Vitamin B_{12} is also often effective.

According to the classic literatures, KIDNEY Meridian passes through throat. So, KI_2 is used at first. I have an experience of a case of severe hoarseness after pneumonectomy. Treatment started over half a year after the operation, but marked improvement was obtained. Effect appeared within several weeks.

[3] Motor Paralysis of Extremities (According to Mr. AOYAGI's oral teaching)
 Sometimes acupuncture is effective for the motor paresis. My standard method is electro-acupuncture selecting points on the meridian that pass the paralyzed muscles and dominating nerves. Supportive use of "Eyelid Acupuncture" is sometimes astonishingly effective.
 It is said that "Eyelid Acupuncture" is a method developed by Mr. PENG Jingshan (Chinese) and Mr. AOYAGI Seidou (Japanese) independently.
 According to their theory, eyelid is divided into 8 zones and 13 sub-segments, and for many diseases, suitable acupuncture treatment is given to suitable segments according to pattern identification. Methods of treatment are scratching, retaining needle or electro-acupuncture etc.
 In my practice, this method is used only for the treatment of motor paralysis. Method of treatment is principally with electro-acupuncture.
 Usually No.20 (0.2mm in diameter) needle 2cm in length is used. Insertion is parallel to the orbital edge about 2mm apart from the margin. Zone "UPPER ENERGIZER (UE)" is used for the upper extremity, and "LOWER ENERGIZER (LE)" is used for the lower extremity. Direction of insertion is not limited, and consideration of supplementation or draining is not necessary. Attention must be paid not to insert whole needle body.

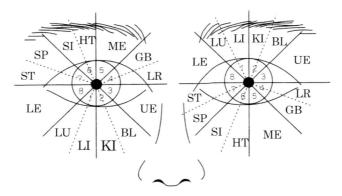

Fig.99 Relation between Segment of Eyelid and ORGANs

 It is difficult to treat both UPPER- and LOWER- ENERGIZER simultaneously. When stimulation of both Energizer point is necessary, one of them must be treated by retaining needle.
 As the vascular network of the face is so rich, that risk of bleeding is not negligible. Enough explanation of the risk must be given before the treatment.
 Frequency of treatment had better to be 2 or 3 times a week. Effect of treatment less than once a week is markedly inferior. The effect of this treatment seems better for the paralysis of the lower extremity.

Motor paralysis of extremities due to brain vascular injury or spinal cord injury is an important subject of rehabilitation. In my practice, such motor paralysis is usually treated with electro-acupuncture of body acupuncture with eyelid acupuncture. Sometimes unexpectedly good effect is obtained. I have an experience of one case of prolonged (over one year from the onset) right hemiplegia. This case showed unexpectedly good effect by this method. It appeared suddenly after treatment several times.

Paralysis of this type often accompanies over-reflection. And not only needle sticking itself is risky, but also risk of intensive involuntary movement caused by electric stimulation or risk of burn by moxa needle are worried. Those who have over-reflection may be contraindication of needle puncture.

Acupuncture for complete anesthetic part is ineffective. However, some patients of cerebrovascular disease feel "Tokki[Jp.] (Getting KI[Jp.])" at needle puncture, and sensation of electric stimulation is left. If hyper-reflection is absent, such cases can be an indication of acupuncture therapy

[4] Myasthenia Gravis

Acupuncture is sometimes effective especially for ocular type.

Detail will be explained later in Chapter 12.

Chapter 4   Acupuncture in Psychiatric Area

Psychosis is extremely distinct medical area, and diagnosis and therapy of psychosis is very difficult for doctors of other area. It should be treated exclusively by psychiatrist.

Acupuncture can remove or decrease many complaints. So, acupuncture is useful in some cases as depressive state and somatoform disorder (psychosomatic disease or general malaise).

§ 1   Depressive State

Real depression is a disease entity, and it should be treated by psychiatrist. However, there are patients of boundary zone, and they are often treated by doctors of other department of medicine. In such case, it is very useful to remove or decrease patient's complaints. They include a lot of symptoms. General fatigue, shoulder stiffness, lumbar pain, headache, complaints of the eye or the throat etc. are often claimed. Kampo$^{(Jp.)}$ formulas are often very effective, and acupuncture is also very useful as previously mentioned. By acupuncture treatment, complaints disappear or decrease, sometimes for long time.

§ 2   Somatoform Disorder

Strong complaints without (or unrelated with) objective findings are often observed. Oriental Medicine is very useful at such "incorporeal" field. As the symptoms, heaviness or pain of the head, shoulder stiffness, lumbar pain, incongruity of the body, anorexia, constipation, incongruity of the throat, symptoms of the eye etc. are often claimed.

For these complaints, Kampo$^{(Jp.)}$ medicine is often used with excellent effects. Acupuncture can treat many of these symptoms and the effects appear very rapidly. Method of the treatment is as mentioned previously. The best way may be collaboration of Kampo medicine and acupuncture.

Sometimes symptoms appear and vanish alternately. In such case, repeating treatment alternately, complaints disappear gradually.

Chapter 5 Diseases of Digestive Organ & Metabolic Diseases

Treatment of this area is performed mainly by Occidental Medicine. For the sedation of abdominal pain, acupuncture is very effective. But, as mentioned before, "sedation of abdominal pain without diagnosis" is very risky. So, the role of acupuncture is attributive in this area.

§ 1 Nausea and Vomiting

Cause of nausea or vomiting is often evident, and the orthodox treatment is to find out its cause and to cure the cause. Treatment only to remove symptom may be wrong. Here, method of Oriental Medicine had better be limited to evidently applicable cases as autointoxication or by the state in which urgent treatment is requested.

Acupuncture is often very effective for nausea &/or vomiting. Usually points of Stomach Meridian (ST), Large Intestine Meridian (LI), Triple Energizer Meridian (TE), Pericardium Meridian (PC) or Conception Vessel (CV) are used for sedating nausea and vomiting. In my experience, the treatment of Spleen Meridian (SP4 or SP3) is the most effective. Acupoint injection is more convenient than electro-acupuncture. Physiological saline solution or vitamin induces good effect. Appearance of effect is very rapid.

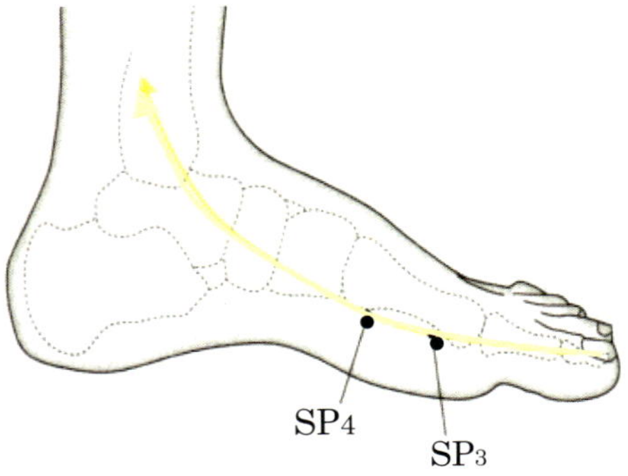

Fig.100 Point for Nausea and Vomiting

§ 2 Hiccup

Hiccup is cramp of the diaphragm via phrenic nerve. Occidental method of the treatment is to paralyze phrenic nerve. It is not so easy, and risk of pneumothorax is not negligible.

In the concept of "FIVE ELEMENT Theory", hiccup is regarded as disease of SOIL. ORGAN of SOIL is STOMACH and SPLEEN. So, as the target of acupuncture therapy of hiccup, STOMACH Meridian (ST) is used. ST$_{34}$, ST$_{36}$, ST$_{41}$, ST$_{43}$ and ST$_{44}$ are often used. Any point is effective, but ST$_{34}$ seems the most effective.

Any method of acupuncture can be used, but acupoint injection is most convenient, because injecting points mentioned above one

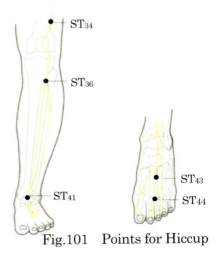

Fig.101 Points for Hiccup

by one, useful point becomes automatically clear. Any substance such as physiological saline solution or vitamins is effective

§ 3 Dehydrated Feeling of the Mouth

Dehydrated feeling of the mouth is often claimed. In many cases, the reason is not clear, and the treatment of the feeling itself is important.

SPLEEN Meridian (SP) spreads under the tongue, KIDNEY Meridian (KI) reaches the root of the tongue, and LIVER Meridian (LR) passes inside of the cheek and the lip.

Treatment of SPLEEN Meridian (SP_3 or SP_4) is very effective. Appearance of the effect is usually very rapid. If the effect is insufficient, point of KIDNEY Meridian (KI_2) &/or Liver Meridian (LR_3 etc.) is added with good effect.

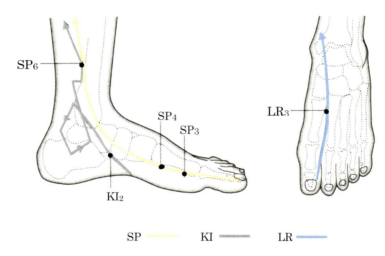

Fig.102 Points for Dehydrated Sensation of Oral Cavity

§ 4 Constipation

Constipation is treated mainly by laxatives, and usually acupuncture has no part to play. In my experience, after injection to LI_4, sometimes obstinate constipation improves. About treatment of postoperative paresis of intestine is mentioned before. For prolonged wind stop due to paresis of intestine after laparotomy, marked accelerating effect of breaking wind often appears by acupoint injection of Vitamin B_1 or B_{12} at LI_4, LI_7 or LI_{10}. Stimulation to point of LARGE INTESTINE Meridian (LI) will stimulate the movement of intestine. Stimulation of finger pressure at LI_4 or LI_{10} sometimes accelerates defecation.

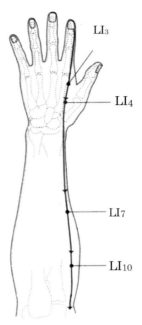

Fig.103 Points for Treatment of Constipation

§ 5 Obesity[24]

The most important key to the treatment of obesity is calorie restriction and movement. And unless the patient has sense of crisis about obesity and hard will to lose weight, successful weight control cannot be performed.

There are some patients who cannot get enough exercise because of the impediment of knee joint etc. Even in such cases, possibility of weight loss remains by some opportunity of small weight loss. Small weight loss often helps subsequent weight loss. Acupuncture is often useful for such cases.

[1] Method of Treatment

Auricular acupuncture with thumbtack needle is used. That is to stick thumbtack needle with very short needle (usually 0.3mm) at suitable place of the auricle, changing it every second week. Many methods are published. In my method, Stomach Point and Hunger Point is used.

Point searching is fairly difficult. Most credible method is to use search meter. Recently fairly economical instrument is available. Painful

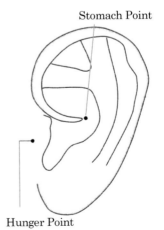

Fig.104 Points of Ear for Treatment of Obesity

point by pressure of handle tip of needle is easy and convenient.

Formerly needle adjusting was difficult. But now, separately sterilized thumbtack needle is available (p.11, p.95), and the problem of adjustment is resolved.

[2] Meal during Treatment

For the treatment of obesity, contents of meal and behavior of eating is very important. Patients have often queer "common sense". For example, not to eat protein (thinking not to take oil and fat), or to eat abundant stir-fried vegetables with much sugar (being convinced that vegetable is useful for weight reducing), or to eat plenty of fruits (convinced that fruits are healthy meal), or to fast in the morning for the weight loss etc. Guidance about these "commonsense" is inevitable.

During the treatment with auricular acupuncture, eating is not limited except sugar and alcohol. It is also important to inhibit snacks between meals.

In many cases, appetite diminishes during treatment. Some patients are anxious about this "anorexia", and make effort to eat much. "To eat according to patient's appetite" is also very important advice.

[3] Process of the Effect

There are various types of process of the effects. The type relatively often observed is that weight loss of 2 or 3 kg appears during the first course of the treatment, and weight loss of 4 to 5 kg is performed after several courses. In many patients, a slight loss of weight gives impetus to further weight loss. Weight loss appears during treatment in some patients, and in some patients it appears after removal of needles. In some patients body weight begins to decrease after the end of treatment. In some patients body weight shows no change, and in some patients body weight increases contrary to expectation.

Generally speaking, a tendency is observed that this method is effective for the really overweight persons. I have an experience that over 20 kilogram's weight loss was achieved for a patient with over 90 kilogram's weight.

[4] Attention by This Treatment

In this treatment, attention must be paid for infection through the course of treatment:

1) Disinfection by Treatment

The auricle skin, except earlobe and "Hunger Point", is closely adhered to cartilage. Cartilage is one of the most sensitive place in the body against infection. So, disinfection is very important.

Disinfection of operation field, especially "Stomach Point", must be done like "a real surgical operation". Usually operation field is wiped with antiseptic swab until the skin is enough clean, and the skin is disinfected with povidone-iodine. Disinfected skin is not decolorized with Hypo Ethanol so as to indicate disinfected area clearly.

Previously, sterilization of needles and putting needle were fairly difficult and troublesome. But now, as separately sterilized thumbtack needle is available, this distress has disappeared (p.11).

After needle pasting, one drip of povidone-iodine is added on the adhesive plaster.

The needles are kept on the ear for one week. Following attentions for patient are very important for the prevention of infection after the treatment.

1. Never wet the ear until the needles are removed (= Never wash hair!).
2. Patients are prohibited to take off needles by themselves.
3. If heat or pain is felt at the ear, patient must visit the practitioner as early as possible.
(If any abnormal findings are found, remove the needle and give antibiotics promptly!)

By removing needle, absence of inflammation must be well checked. It is better to let the patient visit the next day for confirming the absence of inflammation.

2) Follow up after Successful Weight Reducing

This method is useful for reducing body weight itself and also for conditioning to reduce the meal. During treatment and also about one week after removing needles, appetite fairly decreases. Repeating this experience for several weeks, "reducing meal" is conditioned automatically in many patients. If the patient does not keep this custom, body weight will soon, within a few weeks, return to the former level. Education about this phenomenon is very important.

Chapter 6 Diseases of Respiratory Organs

§ 1 Bronchial Asthma

There are several diseases which have similar symptom as bronchial asthma. Now, bronchial asthma is regarded to be a kind of chronic inflammation of the lung, and on the other hand, it has an aspect of allergic disease.

Effectiveness of acupuncture for bronchial asthma is not widely known, but actually its effects are excellent. I cannot imagine the treatment of bronchial asthma without acupuncture.

Bronchial asthma is a disease of the lung. Regardless of whether LUNG of Oriental Medicine is equal to the anatomical lung of Occidental Medicine, the both has some similarity. For the treatment of bronchial asthma, point on LUNG Meridian (mainly LU_7, sometimes LU_6 especially for moxa needle) is used.

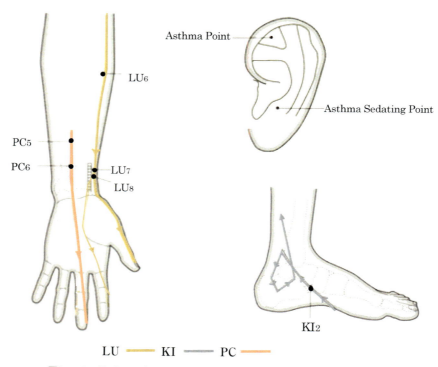

Fig.105 Points for treatment of Bronchial Asthma

Bronchial asthma has an aspect of allergic disease that has close relation with adrenal body and thymus. From this point of view, points of KIDNEY Meridian (mainly KI_2) and PERICARDIUM Meridian (mainly PC_5) are used.

This factor will be mentioned in Chapter 12.

The treatment of KIDNEY Meridian seems most effective for the complaints of bronchial asthma. It may be owing to the following reasons.

- According to the classic literatures, KIDNEY Meridian enters into LUNG and goes upwards alongside trachea.
- Bronchial asthma is a disease of "WATER". "KIDNEY" dominates "WATER".
- Usually the patient feels strongest distress at the sternal region where KIDNEY Meridian (KI) passes.

These factors may be the reason of special effect of KIDNEY Meridian (KI). By the treatment of KIDNEY Meridian alone, asthma attach is often relieved promptly.

Prophylactic effect is also observed. I have an experience that incidentally given moxa needle to KI_2 (for a patient of lumbar pain) induced remarkable effect for the bronchial asthma suffering for many years.

The method of treatment is principally electro-acupuncture. For acute attack, acupoint injection is very useful. With any substances as vitamins or saline solution, excellent effects appear promptly. Together with the intravenous injection of theophylline, the effect is more evident, so as not inferior to drip infusion of corticosteroids

The relation with PERICARDIUM MERIDIAN (PC) will be mentioned later in Chapter 12.

§ 2 Diseases with Asthma-like Symptom

There are some diseases which have toss and dyspnea like bronchial asthma such as cardiac asthma, COPD, emphysema, reflux esophagitis, tuberculosis etc.

For these diseases, acupuncture (including acupoint injection) is effective for cough and dyspnea by the same method of acupuncture treatment for bronchial asthma. But the duration of the effect is usually short, at most one or two days. If acupuncture is not effective for "asthma", it is better to search other origin of cough &/or dyspnea

Chapter 7   Acupuncture in Gynecology

§ 1   Dysmenorrhea

Some patients with dysmenorrhea, such as endometriosis, must be treated by Occidental Medicine. However, "to remove patients' present suffering" is also important therapy, including the case of endometriosis etc. For this purpose, Kampo(Jp.) medicine is a kind of radical therapy and it is very effective. But selection of formula is not so easy, and its effects do not appear promptly.

Effecs of acupuncture therapy appear rapidly. In almost all cases, patients' complaints of dysmenorrhea disappear promptly. Treatment is necessary only once for one menstruation. Meridian & point selection is much easier than selection of Kampo(Jp.) formula. So, acupuncture is very useful for the treatment of dysmenorrhea.

Acupoint injection is also effective as electro-acupuncture. With acupoint injection, neither diagnosis of deficiency-or-excess of meridians nor consideration of supplementation or draining of therapy is necessary, and it is not always essential to hit point exactly. So, even a beginner who has almost no knowledge of acupuncture can practice this method as far as the practitioner is authorized to give injection. Pharmacologically inactive substances such as saline solution or vitamin can produce excellent effect. Thumbtack needle is also effective.

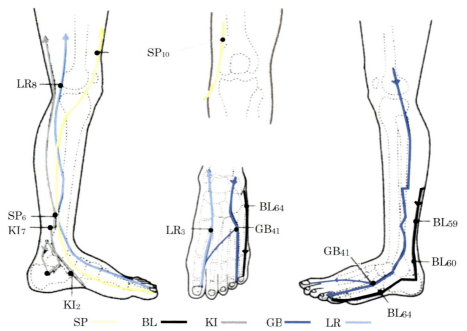

Fig.106   Points for Treatment of Dysmenorrhea

Method is as described below by any method of acupuncture.
1. **Fundamental point selection**:
    SPLEEN-Meridian: SP_6 or SP_{10}
    KIDNEY Meridian: KI_2 or KI_7
    LIVER Meridian: LR_3 or LR_8
    Excellent effects appear very often with only one treatment of bilateral SP_6 or SP_{10}. Then farther treatment is not necessary.
2. If **lumber pain** is combined, treatment of BL_{59} or BL_{60} and GB_{35} is added.
3. If **nausea** is combined, and treatment of SP_6 or SP_{10} is ineffective, treatment of SP_4 is added.

By acupoingt injection, the order of the treatment is:
SP_6 (or SP_{10}) → KI_7 or KI_2 → LR_8 → KI_2 → LR_3 → BL_{59} or BL_{60} → GB_{35}
   ↑   (For Lumber Pain)
If not enough effective, according to the symptom ⎦
When enough effect appears, farther treatment is not necessary.

§ 2   Menopausal Disorder

Symptoms of menopausal disorder are diverse, and often various symptoms appear one after another. Occidental Medicine is not always definitely effective. Kampo(Jp.) medicine is often very effective, but selection of the formulas is not so easy and effects do not appear promptly.

Acupuncture may not be a radical treatment, but it is useful for reduction of complaints. Removing each complaint one by one, the patient is often gradually relieved from complaints completely. The method of treatment for each complaint is mentioned before. Using suitable Kampo(Jp.) formula together, better effect is expected.

§ 3   Emesis (Morning Sickness)

Emesis (morning sickness) is one of the hardest complications of pregnancy. It happens at the earliest stage of pregnancy, and at this stage, fetus is very sensitive for medication and radiation.

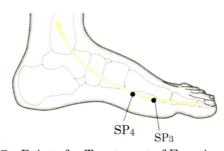

Fig.107   Points for Treatment of Emesis

My first experience was 28y.o. pregnant woman suffering from severest nausea. Just after injection of saline solution to bilateral SP$_4$ 0.1ml each, she cried "Ah I feel hungry!". After 2 weeks, she felt slight nausea again, and by the same treatment, she has recovered completely from morning sickness. Thereafter several cases were treated in the same way (including electro-acupuncture), and it was very effective for all patients. Duration of effect is various. In most of cases, the effects continue more than 1week.

When the treatment of SPLEEN Meridian is not effective enough, adding treatment of STOMACH Meridian (ST$_{36}$, ST$_{34}$ etc.), effects are often widely promoted.

§ 4 Painless Delivery

There are many reports of painless delivery with acupuncture. I tried it with electro-acupuncture several times, but it was not successive. Pain surely decreases, but labor decreases simultaneously.

In experience of premedication for laparotomy, acupoint injection may be useful for the painless delivery. Using pharmacologically inactive substances for slight pain and using strong analgesics as Pentazocine for strong pain, painless delivery may be successfully performed.

Chapter 8   Acupuncture in Dermatology

§ 1   General Rule for Acupuncture for Dermal Disease

There is a concept in Oriental Medicine that "Skin and hair belong to LUNG". Function of LUNG is not entirely equal to the function of the lung, but taking into consideration that swimming or rubdown with a dry towel is adopted in the treatment of asthma, this concept may not be regarded nonsensical. Anyway, treatment on points of LUNG Meridian (LU) for skin diseases very often induces excellent effects.

Principally, for the treatment of skin diseases, invariably points of LUNG Meridian (LU) are used according to the classic literatures. Often treatment is completed by the treatment of LUNG Meridian (LU) only, but combined with treatment on points of meridians that pass through the area of the lesion, effect is more evident.

The order of treatment is:

① Point of LUNG Meridian (LU_7 or LU_6 or LU_8) is treated independent of the location of the lesion (except Herpes Zoster).

② The prioritization of other meridian selection is:
  1. Parts of subjectively strong distress.
  2. Parts of prominent lesion
  3. Patient's worrying parts
  4. Other parts if it is necessary

As the method of treatment, electro-acupuncture is most frequently used, but thumbtack needle or acupoint injection is also useful. These methods are often used together.

For the treatment of skin diseases, Kampo[Jp.] medicine is often very effective. Meanwhile acupuncture is competent to remove subjective distress. So, as the treatment of skin diseases by Oriental Medicine, often Kampo medicine plays the leading role and acupuncture is used as supporting role for the treatment of distress. In the same meaning, collaboration of Occidental Medicine and acupuncture is also useful. Owing to the use of acupuncture, often reduction or withdrawal of steroid hormone is succeeded.

In many kinds of dermal diseases, allergy or immunity are concerned. So, KIDNEY Meridian and PERICARDIUM Meridian are used together. This factor will be mentioned in Chapter 12.

Lesion of skin is visible. So, by most cases, effect can be objectively estimated except grade of itch and pain.

§ 2 Urticaria

Method of treatment of urticaria is established in Occidental Medicine. But drowsiness by antihistaminic drugs is often inconvenient for daily life. Acupuncture has no such side effect, and sometimes it causes excellent effect.

Any methods of acupuncture are usable, but acupoint injection is most convenient and effective. Mostly urticaria appears in whole body. But independent of the location of lesion, treatment of only LUNG Meridian (LU) is often very effective. Pharmacologically inactive medicine as saline solution or vitamins is enough effective. Mostly LU_7 is used. In most cases, itch sensation disappears promptly at a single injection. Sometimes exanthema diminishes or disappears. Usually disappearance of exanthema delays, but by disappearance of itch sensation, "purpose of the treatment" is mostly achieved. Compared with antihistaminic drugs, effect and durability of acupuncture is somewhat inferior. But in regard to rapid appearance of effect and no side effects, acupuncture is superior to drugs.

§ 3 Erosion around Artificial Anus

Erosion often appears around the artificial anus, and it is painful and very refractory, and its handling often troubles doctors and nurses. Acupuncture is useful for this lesion. For the relief of the pain, acupoint injection with vitamins etc. is enough useful. For the treatment of erosion, electro-acupuncture is better.

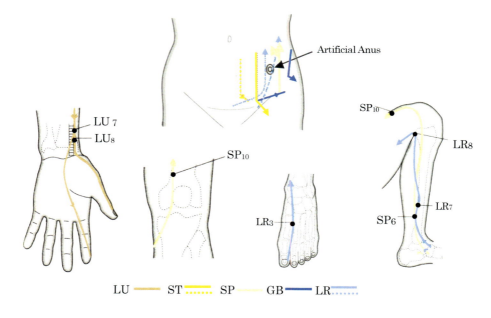

Fig.108 Meridians around Usual Artificial Anus and Points of Treatment

Artificial anus is usually set at the left lower abdomen where LIVER Meridian (LR) and SPLEEN Meridian pass. So, points of LUNG Meridian (LU$_7$), SPLEEN Meridian (SP$_6$ or SP$_{10}$) and LIVER Meridian (LR$_3$ or LR$_5$ or LR$_8$) are treated. With acupoint injection, injection to LU$_7$ and SP$_6$ often causes excellent effect for pain sedation

§ 4 Fresh Herpes Zoster

The most important problem of Herpes Zoster is pain. Neuralgic pain as sequela of Herpes Zoster is mentioned before (p.176). It is purely problem of neural injury.

As visual lesion of Herpes Zoster is usually flamboyant, patients (often as well as doctors) focus exclusively on the lesion of the skin, and not on reducing the pain.

Recently medications that are effective against Herpes Zoster virus have been developed. They are useful for curing the lesion or reduction of suffering time, but it is not always effective for lessening the pain. Prophylaxis of PHN by these medications is not sure. On the other hand, exanthema surely heals without any treatments, sometimes regardless of inadequate bad treatment. So, it may be no exaggeration to say that the most important treatment of Herpes Zoster is pain control. Some say that Herpes Zoster is a disease of anesthesiology.

As a measure of pain relief, nerve block is often used, and acupuncture is also a strong method of pain control. I cannot imagine "treatment without acupuncture" for Herpes Zoster

In treatment of Herpes Zoster, treatment of pain should be mainly taken into consideration. "Treatment exclusively considering pain relief" seems to produce excellent effect also for the cure of lesion of the skin lesion.

[1] Method of treatment

Both electro-acupuncture and acupoint injection are used. For acupoint injection, considering pharmacological effect, vitamin B$_{12}$ is mostly used. Its effect is also excellent like electro-acupuncture. It is not inadequate to treat mild Herpes Zoster with acupoint injection and examine the relation between points and effect. But as the treatment of Herpes Zoster must be given frequently and sometimes for a long time, electro-acupuncture is more convenient, and the effect of electro-acupuncture seems to be better than acupoint injection. Seeing the progress of the effect of acupoint injection for a few weeks, if the effect is insufficient, it is better to change method of treatment into electro-acupuncture.

[2] Meridian & Point Selection

As the location of exanthema & pain is almost always the same, meridian selection is easy. If the location of each is not matched, location of the pain should be selected. It is inadequate to use points at the part of exanthema because the place of exanthema is extremely sensitive for pain. In the extremities, it is often difficult to find intact place, and sometimes it is necessary to use points at the trunk or the head.

In the case of the intercostal region, pain and exanthema extend to broad area, and the practitioner is often at a loss about meridian selection. In such case, meridian is selected as intercostal neuralgia (p.176), and the order of meridian selection is decided according to the strength of the pain.

For the patients with pain of the eye such as corneal herpes, treatment of LR_3 is effective. If it is very severe, treatment of CONCEPTION VESSEL (CV_{22}) &/or "Eye Point" in the auricle together with LR_3 is recommended. For Ramsey-Hunt's Syndrome, treatment of ST_{43} or ST_{44}, TE_2 or TE_3 and LR_3 is effective. If the taste disorder is accompanied, adding the treatment of SP_4, excellent effects are obtained.

Treatment of the points of LUNG Meridian (LU), which is basic method for skin diseases, is not effective for the pain of Herpes Zoster, except the lesion at the LUNG Meridian (LU) region.

[3] **Effect of Acupuncture and the Course**

Effects of acupuncture for the fresh Herpes Zoster is excellent. Especially by electro-acupuncture, complete cure is surely obtained without leaving neuralgia, so long as the treatment is correctly continued.

Course of the effect of acupuncture therapy for Herpes Zoster is distinct. By electro-acupuncture as well as acupoint injection, pain decreases at the beginning of the treatment. Sometimes the pain disappears completely. However, the pain usually reappears after 30 minutes to 3 hours, and the patient often feels stronger than before treatment, probably due to the contrast phenomenon. Thereafter pain decreases gradually within one or two days (Fig.109). There is almost no exception. This phenomenon should be well explained to the patient and the family before the treatment. Patients often discontinue acupuncture therapy by lack of the knowledge of this phenomenon, supposing that the effect is only temporal. Rebound just after the acupuncture is the most troublesome problem on fresh Herpes Zoster.

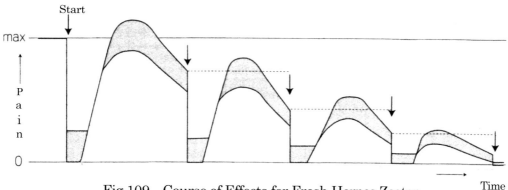

Fig.109   Course of Effects for Fresh Herpes Zoster

[4] Frequency and Length of Treatment

The frequency of the treatment is "the more frequent the better". Between less than once a week and once a week, serious difference of effect is observed. The difference of effect between once a week and twice a week is also remarkable. The difference between twice a week and thrice a week, some difference of the effect is observed, but not always. It is desirable to treat at least twice a week.

Necessary length of the treatment varies. In some cases pain disappears by only one treatment. And some cases it requires very long period. It depends on the frequency of treatment to some extent. Remained pain after one month from the onset of the disease should be treated as before mentioned PHN.

§ 5　Atopic Dermatitis

There are many methods of treatment in Occidental Medicine for atopic dermatitis. Oriental Medicine is also effective. Kampo$^{(Jp.)}$ medicine is sometimes very effective without side effects. Here acupuncture cannot play leading role, but sometimes it is very useful.

One of the causes of disease progression is scratching due to itch sensation. By "reduce itch sensation for decrease scratching", the lesion promotes remarkably. For this purpose, "treatment of LUNG Meridian (LU)" mentioned before is very useful. Treatment of LU$_7$ or LU$_6$ is convenient, but by point selection attention is necessary about deviation of the point by position of the arm (p.49).

Here intradermal acupuncture (including thumbtack needle) is most convenient. In almost all cases, just after pricking LU$_7$, itch sensation decreases markedly or sometimes disappears.

Direction of puncture is "along-or-against the flow" of meridian according to deficiency-or-excess of pulse diagnosis. By reverse estimation of this relation, often opposite effect appears immediately. But correction is easy by sticking needle into reverse direction. Putting vertical direction (as by Thumbtack needle) is also effective. Needle insertion technique and adjustment of intradermal acupuncture is a little difficult. Thumbtack needle is technically easier and also effective. But for some patients who have very narrow range of point, hitting exact point is fairly difficult without search meter (p.85).

Atopic dermatitis has a close relation with immunity. So, KIDNEY Meridian (usually KI$_2$) and PERICARDIUM Meridian (usually PC$_5$) are always used. This will be explained again in Chapter 12.

§ 6　Palmoplantar Pustulosis

Palmoplantar Pustulosis is an intractable disease, but acupuncture therapy is very effective. It has close relation with allergy or immunity.

Treatment of this disease will be explained again in Chapter 12.

Chapter 9   Acupuncture for Complaints of Ear, Nose and Throat

§ 1   Acupuncture for Disorder of the Ear

[1] Meridians and Points Related to the Ear

In general meridian charts, SMALL INTESTINE Meridian (SI), TRIPLE ENERGIZER Meridian (TE) and GALLBLADDER Meridian (GB) arrive near the ear. According to the classic literatures, SI-meridian and TE-Meridian enter into the ear, and a branch of GB-Meridian enters into the ear dividing from GB_{20}. KIDNEY is regarded to have close relation with the ear. ("KIDNEY opens at the ear").

For auricular acupuncture, "Inner Ear", "Middle Ear" and "External Ear" are indicated. Middle Ear and External Ear are not easy to use.

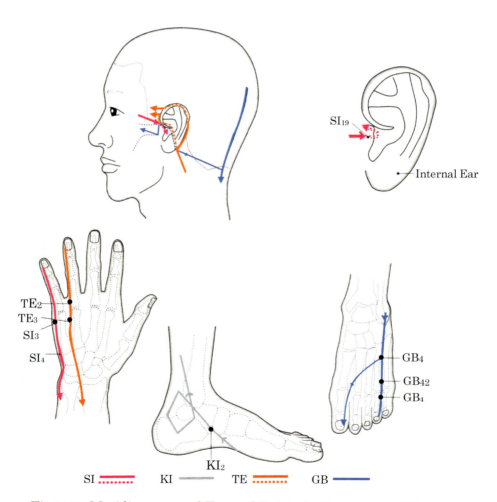

Fig.110   Meridians around Ear and Points for Symptoms of Ear

[2] Pain of the Ear

For the treatment of pain, points of SMALL INTESTINE Meridian (SI₃ orSI₆), TRIPLE ENERGIZER Meridian (TE₂ or TE₃) and Gallbladder Meridian (GB₄₁ or GB₄₂ or GB₄₃) are used. With any method of acupuncture, excellent effect is obtained. By acupoint injection with strong analgesics as Pentazocine, severest pain can be sedated.

[3] Tinnitus, Dizziness, Hearing Loss

These symptoms are trouble of the inner ear. But Oriental Medicine has other distinct idea as described below.

1) These symptoms are regarded as "WATER Poisoning".
2) According to "Five Element Theory", dizziness belongs to the disease of "WOOD".

Considering these theories, points of KIDNEY Meridian (mainly KI₂) and Gallbladder Meridian (mainly GB₄₃) are often used together.

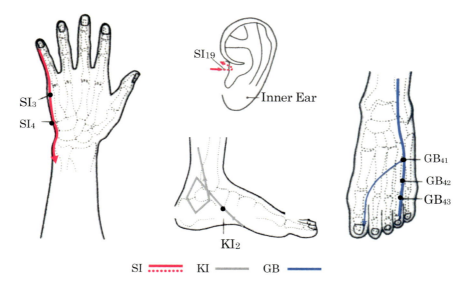

Fig111   Points for Treatment of Tinnitus, Dizziness & Deafness

A. Hearing Loss
1. Conductive Hearing Loss

Effects of acupuncture for deafness are not sure, but sometimes it is unexpectedly effective. Sometimes inflammation is related with conductive hearing loss. Possibly good effect may be expected for some patients, owing to the effect of acupuncture for inflammation.

Method of treatment is usually electro-acupuncture. For the treatment, points of SMALL INTESTINE Meridian (SI), TRIPLE ENERGIZER Meridian (TE) and

GALLBLADDER Meridian (GB) are selected. If KIDNEY Meridian (KI) is deficient, moxa needle is added to KI$_2$. As auricular acupuncture, "Inner Ear" point is used. Frequently used points are:

SMALL INTESTINE Meridian: SI$_3$ or SI$_4$
  SI$_{19}$ is used according to the mutual patient's consent.
TRIPLE ENERGIZER Meridian: TE$_2$ or TE$_3$
GALLBLADDER Meridian: GB$_{43}$
KIDNEY Meridian: KI$_2$
Auricle: Inner Ear Point

2. Sensorineural Hearing Loss

Hearing loss of this type is regarded as "WATER Poisoning" in Oriental Medicine. Usual method of treatment is:

Electro-acupuncture:
  Inner Ear Point of auricle
  TRIPLE ENERGIZER (mainly TE$_3$)
    or SMALL INTESTINE Meridian (SI$_3$ or SI$_{19}$)
  KIDNEY Meridian (mainly KI$_2$)
Moxa needle:
  SMALL INTESTINE Meridian (SI$_3$)
    or TRIPLE ENERGIZER Meridian (TE$_3$)
  GALLBLADDER Meridian (GB$_{41}$ or GB$_{43}$)

Effect of acupuncture for inner ear hearing loss is uncertain, but sometimes it is unexpectedly effective for senile deafness.

B. Tinnitus

Tinnitus is a problem of the inner ear. In Oriental Medicine, tinnitus is regarded as "WATER poisoning" which has a close relation with KIDNEY. Considering this factor, together with the relation between the ear and meridians, points of SMALL INTESTINE Meridian (SI), TRIPLE ENERGIZER Meridian (TE), GALLBLADDER Meridian (GB), KIDNEY Meridian (KI) and Inner Ear Point of the auricle are used for the treatment of tinnitus. Point selection is similar to the points of sensorineural hearing loss. Method of treatment is mainly electro-acupuncture and moxa needle. Thumbtack needle is used as supplementary measure. Namely, electro-acupuncture is used at Point of Inner Ear of auricle, TE$_3$ and KI$_2$, and moxa needle is added to SI$_3$ and GB$_{41}$ or GB$_{43}$. After this treatment, thumbtack needle is put at these points.

Effect for tinnitus is extremely different according to the origin. Effects for tinnitus associated with whiplash syndrome is usually excellent, but effect for tinnitus due to sudden deafness is almost ineffective. For senile tinnitus, acupuncture is usually ineffective without rare exception.

C. Dizziness

There are several primary diseases of dizziness other than labyrinthine origin. In Oriental Medicine, dizziness is regarded as "WATER Poisoning", and according to "Five Element Theory" it is a disease of "WOOD System (GALLBLADDER and LIVER)". Treatment of acupuncture for dizziness is also independent of the origin.

Methods are mainly electro-acupuncture using point of Inner Ear of auricle, KIDNEY Meridian (KI$_2$) and GALLBLADDER Meridian (GB$_{41}$ or GB$_{43}$). According to my experience, electric stimulation for TE$_3$ by whiplash injury was very effective for dizziness, if pulse diagnosis is deficient, moxa needle for TE$_3$ is added.

Effects for dizziness are also extremely different according to the origin. Effect of dizziness by whiplash injury is excellent. For the most of them, treatment of auricle point is not necessary. For dizziness by vertebra-basilar insufficiency, acupuncture is almost ineffective. Effect for rotary vertigo such as so called Meniere's syndrome is often excellent, but treatment for dizziness as wobbly or floating or as if sinking etc. is rarely effective. If nausea is accompanied with dizziness, treatment (acupoint injection or moxa needle) for SP$_4$ is very effective even if treatment for dizziness is ineffective (p.185)

[4] Symptoms of the Nose

According to general meridian charts, LARGE INTESTINE Meridian (LI) and GOVERNOR VESSEL (GV) are related with the nose, and BLADDER Meridian starts near the root of the nose. According to classic literatures, STOMACH Meridian (ST) starts from inside of the nose. Almost all the complaints of nose are solved by acupuncture treatment of LARGE INTESTINE Meridian (usually LI$_4$ or LI$_{10}$) and STOMACH Meridian (usually ST$_{43}$ or ST$_{44}$).

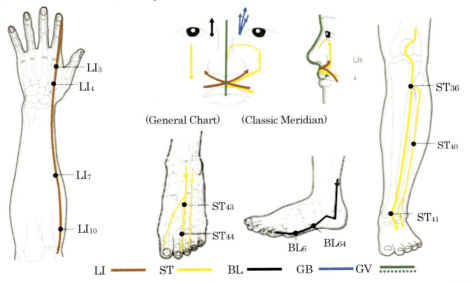

Fig.112 Meridians around Nose and Points for Treatment of Complaints of Nose

Any methods of acupuncture are possible for the treatment of the nose. Thumbtack needle is useful for prolongation of the effect. Meridian-and-point selection is independent of the origin of complaints, but if it is connected with allergy, point of KIDNEY Meridian (usually KI$_2$) and PERICARDIUM Meridian (PC$_3$ or PC$_6$) are treated together.

[5] Pollinosis

Pollinosis is a good indication of acupuncture. It is easily cured by acupuncture and Kampo$^{(Jp.)}$ medicine. Method will be explained in Chapter 12.

[6] Complaints of Pharyngo-Laryngeal Region

In general meridian charts, only CONCEPTION VESSEL (CV) passes this area. But according to the classic literature, many meridians pass through this area as described below.

SPLEEN Meridian (SP) passes through the throat and the root of the tongue, and spreads under the tongue.

HEART Meridian (HT): One branch passes the throat and reaches the eye.

KIDNEY Meridian (KI) goes upward along the trachea, passes the throat and reaches CV$_{23}$ via the root of the tongue.

LIVER Meridian passes the larynx and reaches GV$_{20}$ via the eye.

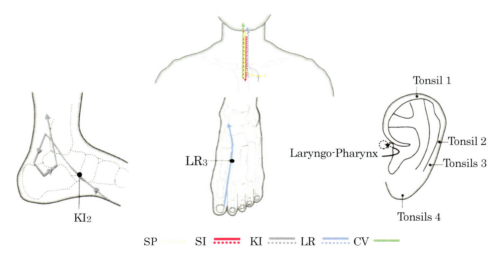

Fig.113 Meridians of Pharyngo-Laryngeal region and Points for Treatment

Treatment of laryngeal pain is mentioned in Chapter 1. For the pain of tonsillitis, swallowing after gargle of Kanzoutou $^{(Jp.)}$ (Gan-cao Tang$^{(Ch.)}$, a Kampo medicine), is very effective. If this treatment is not effective enough, the pain can be sedated by acupoint injection to KI$_2$. Any substance as saline solution or vitamin is effective. Antibiotics are almost unnecessary.

Among four meridians mentioned above, KIDNEY Meridian (KI) is mainly used. Almost all symptoms of pharynx can be relieved by treatment of KI$_2$ (by acupoint injection or electro-acupuncture) as mentioned before.

There is a point of auricle "Throat". But it is very inconvenient to use. There are points of "Tonsils" in the auricle, but it is rarely used.

Chapter 10 Acupuncture in Ophthalmology

§ 1 General Rule

In general meridian charts, BLADDER Meridian (BL) and GALLBLADDER Meridian pass near the eye. According to the classic literatures, many meridians are in a close relation with the eye as described below.

HEART Meridian (HT): One branch connects with the eye passing through the throat.

SMALL INTESTINE Meridian (SI): One branch goes to the medial ocular angle.

BLADDER Meridian (BL) starts from the medial ocular angle.

TRIPLE ENERGIZER Meridian (TE): One branch reaches lateral end of the eyebrow via the lateral ocular angle, and another branch passes behind the auricle and reaches the zygomatic bone via frontal region and the medial ocular angle.

GALLBLADDER Meridian (GB) starts from the outside of lateral ocular angle, and one branch goes to the eye via the lower jaw.

LIVER Meridian (LR) goes to GV_{20} passing through the eye.

CONCEPTION VESSEL (CV) enters the eye after passing around the lip.

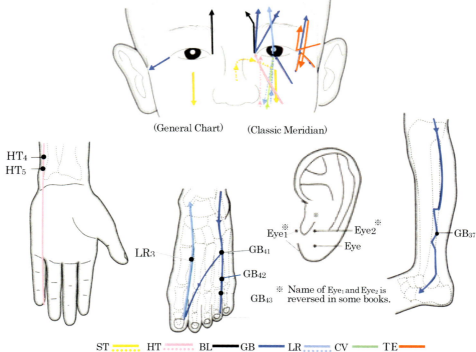

Fig.114 Meridians around Eye and Points for Treatment of Complaints of Eye

Among these meridians, LIVER Meridian (mostly LR$_3$) is most frequently used, and sometimes HEART Meridian (HT$_4$ or HT$_5$) and CONCEPTION VESSEl (mostly CV$_{22}$) are used. There are three points of the eye in the auricle. They are "Eye", "Eye$_1$" and "Eye$_2$". The meaning is not clear, and the naming "Eye$_1$" and "Eye$_2$" is lack of unity between books. By the electro-acupuncture of auricular point, short needle is inserted from "Eye" point to rear "Eye$_2$" (of Fig.114). But auricular acupuncture is seldom necessary. Here acupoint injection is possible.

In many cases, by the treatment of GALLBLADDER Meridian (GB$_{35}$, GB$_{41}$, GB$_{42}$ or GB$_{43}$ etc.), patients often say that "Visual field became lighter". Sometimes by treatment of these points, complaints of eye disappear without aiming it.

Ophthalmology is an extremely specialized area. So, as if patient's complaint disappeared by acupuncture therapy, attention should be paid not to interrupt the treatment of ophthalmologist.

§ 2 Pain of the Eye

Pain of the eye is often complained. But its origin is not always at the eye. But the method of acupuncture treatment is always the same, independent of the origin of the cause. In almost all cases, treatment of LR$_3$ is effective enough. If pain remains and its origin is not clear, treatment must be trusted to ophthalmologist.

§ 3 Diplopia

Acupuncture therapy is sometimes effective for diplopia of the myasthenia gravis and diplopia after a traffic accident. Principle of treatment is as mentioned in § 1. Usually points of meridians that pass around injured muscle. For example, points of BLADDER Meridian (mainly BL$_{64}$) for internal strabismus, and GALLBLADDER Meridian (GB$_{41}$ or GB$_{43}$) &/or TRIPLE ENERGIZER Meridian (TE$_2$ or TE$_3$) etc. for divergent strabismus. Combined treatment of CV$_{22}$ &/or Eye Points of ear lobe is often very useful.

According to my experience, acupoint injection is sometimes effective for diplopia after traffic accident. Effect of acupoint injection appears soon after the injection. So, the points to be treated become promptly clear by the effect of acupoit injection. Duration of the effect is often insufficient.

§ 4 Ocular Hypertension

There is no case of acupuncture treatment with the aim of treatment of ocular hypertension. According to my experience, by some patients, ocular hypertension decreased after effective treatment of the complaints of the eye. In such case, the patient tends to trust acupuncture too strongly, and sometimes relies treatment of the eye on acupuncture. It is not desirable, and it is important to let such patient continue ophthalmologist's therapy.

Chapter 11 Acupuncture for Urinary Organ and Impotence

One case of surprisingly effective IgA nephropathy was experienced. It will be presented in Chapter 12. For other cases of this area, effect of acupuncture seems inferior to Occidental Medicine or Kampo$^{(Jp.)}$ medicine. But it does not mean acupuncture is useless. It is helpful for some cases.

§ 1   Dysuria

KIDNEY and LIVER have close relation with urogenital organs. According to this concept, points of KIDNEY Meridian (KI$_2$ or KI$_7$) and LIVER Meridian (LR$_3$ or LR$_8$) are treated for dysuria, and as SPLEEN Meridian has close relation with these two meridians, SP$_6$ is often used together. Acupoint injection is also effective. Any substances as saline solution or vitamin are available.

It is sometimes fairly effective for dysuria due to prostatic hypertrophy, prostatitis or postoperative dysuria.

§ 2   Urolithiasis

Urolithiasis therapy is established in Occidental Medicine, and "treatment by acupuncture" may be meaningless. But for some cases of pain by "stone attack" acupuncture is effective. Acupoint injection with analgesics as Pentazocine is most convenient and effective. For associated nausea, injection to SP$_4$ is effective. Medication of antispasmodic drug together is desirable.

§ 3   Impotence

Some patients of whiplash syndrome claim impotence. In this case, as an object of main treatment is stiffness of the neck & the shoulder, headache or numbness of the arm etc., treatment for impotence is restricted. Usually moxa needle is used at SP$_6$. Often good result is obtained by this simple method. There are many methods of acupuncture treatment for impotence. But, effect of the treatment for other type of impotence is poor with my method.

§ 4   IgA Nephropathy

This will be mentioned in the next chapter.

Chapter 12 Allergic or Autoimmune Disorders

§ 1 General Rule

Recently, immunology has marvelously advanced. Diagnosis and therapy of diseases related with allergy or autoimmunity is making rapid progress. Especially improvement of molecular targeted therapy is remarkable. However, catastrophic medical cost and side effects of new therapies may be not negligible.

Treatment of acupuncture is effective for some allergic diseases and autoimmune diseases with low cost and without side effects. In this category, many experiences of excellent effects were obtained under the basic concept of my acupuncture. A kind of innovation of the idea of immunology may be achieved under my method.

From the early period of starting acupuncture, I doubted equality of ORGAN in Oriental Medicine and organ in Occidental Medicine. ORGAN in Oriental Medicine seemed me to be a concept which has both morphological and functional aspects. From that point of view, some ORGANs are very similar to other organs of Occidental Medicine with different anatomical name as described below.

1. Function of **SPLEEN** is not that of spleen, but it seems almost equal to the function of **pancreas**. In Spanish speaking world, SPLEEN Meridian is called "Meridiano vazo-pancreatico (Spleno-pancreatic Meridian"). That seems me very reasonable.
2. Function of **KIDNEY** is not of kidney. Its function seems just function of **adrenal body**.
3. According to the description of the classic literature[8] of **PERICARDIUM**, its role is to guard HEART and it is provided shape of network. This description actually implicates **thymus** as the corresponding organ.

Thymus produces T-cell, and it is regarded to be the center of immunity. From adrenal medulla, adrenaline (which is used by allergic shock at first) is secreted, and from adrenal cortex, cortical hormones which are widely used for the treatment of allergic diseases and autoimmune diseases.

From these points of view, for the treatment of diseases which is related with immunity, points of KIDNEY Meridian (usually KI$_2$) and PERICARDIUM Meridian (usually PC$_5$) are selected at first, and then points according to the symptoms are selected. The reason to select KI$_2$ is, because it is easiest to use in the KIDNEY Meridian, and it seems most effective in my impression. PC$_5$ and PC$_6$ are regarded to have close relation with LUNG Meridian (LU) & HEART Meridian (HT) which have often close relation with targeted diseases. Both PC$_5$ and PC$_6$ are situated at tendon-rich area, but tendons are rather sparser around PC$_5$. That is why I select PC$_5$ rather than PC$_6$. Some of these diseases are already mentioned before, but I would like to explain here again in a lump.

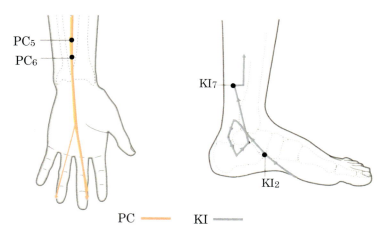

Fig.115 Fundamental Points for Autoimmune Disease

§ 2 Bronchial Asthma (cf. Chapter6 §1)

By the attack of bronchial asthma, usually patients complain strongest anguish at the sternal region where KIDNEY Meridian passes. The first experience of acupuncture treatment for bronchial asthma was acupoint injection to LU_7 and KI_2 with vitamin B_1, for a patient of status asthmaticus. It was surprisingly effective. After several years, treatment of PC_5 and KI_2 started for diseases related with allergy. Now point selection for the treatment of bronchial asthma is LU_7, KI_2 and PC_5. Effect is not evidently different from treatment of LU_7 and KI_2, but duration of effect seems elongated. Using intravenous use of aminophylline together, the effect seems to be equal to (sometimes better than) drip infusion of corticosteroid hormone.

This treatment is effective also for asthma-like diseases as cardiac asthma etc. But duration of effect for other diseases is evidently shorter. It seems to be a proof of the effect of KI_2 and PC_5 for diseases related with allergy or immunity.

§ 3 Pollinosis (Allergic Rhinitis and Conjunctivitis)

Main symptoms of pollinosis are sneezing, rhinorrhea, nasal obstruction and itching of the eye. Kampo(Jp.) medicines are very effective for the treatment and prevention. But its effect does not appear promptly, and selection of formula is not so easy. Acupuncture is superior at the point of easy application and rapid appearance of effect without any side effect except pain from needing or injection.

According to classic literatures, main meridians related with the nose are LARGE INTESTINE Meridian (LI) and STOMACH Meridian (ST), and main meridians related

Chapter 12 Allergic or Autoimmune Disorders 211

with the eye are LIVER Meridian (LR) and CONCEPTION VESSEL (CV). Treatment of LR3 is always excellent for complaints of the eye. So, for the treatment of pollinosis, LR3, LI4 and ST43 or ST44 were used with excellent effect.

Later, adding treatment of KI2 and PC5, effect has evidently improved. Direct effects are not so different, but duration of effect became much longer. Usually Kampo(Jp.) medicine is used together with acupuncture. So, exact comparison is difficult. But frequency and total count of treatment decreased markedly (often Kampo medicine became unnecessary). Many patients who were treated successfully with acupuncture, symptoms in the follwing year become much slighter. Such patients increased by new method.

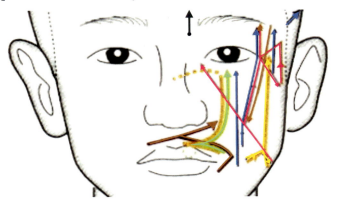

Fig.116-1 Classic Meridians around Nose and Eye

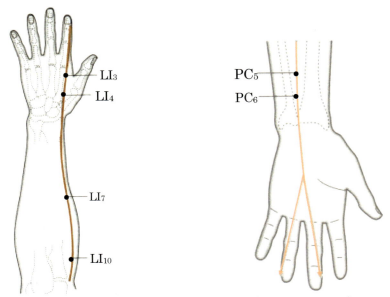

Fig.116-2 Points for Treatment of Pollinosis (Arm and Hand)

LI —— ST —— SI ······· TE —— GB —— CV —— PC ——

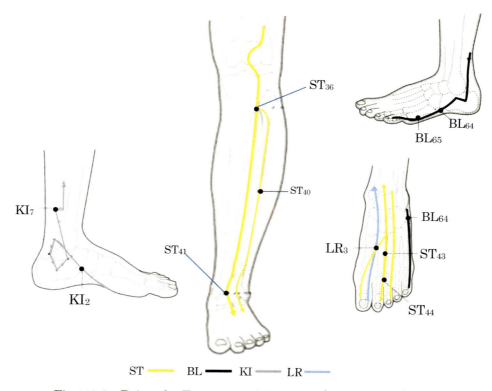

Fig.116-3 Points for Treatment of Pollinosis (Leg and Foot)

My point selection for electro-acupuncture is KI_2, PC_5 and one of LR_3 or LI_4 (or ST_{43} or ST_{44}) for electric stimulation, and moxa needle for other two or three of LR_3 or LI_4 (&/or ST_{43} or ST_{44}).

Selection is due to the heaviness of complaint of the nose and the eye. If the complaint of the eye is more severe, LR_3 is stimulated by electricity and vice versa. Selection of LI_4 and ST_{43} or ST_{44} for electric stimulation is according to usability.

Acupoint injection is very convenient to use. With any substances such as saline solution etc. excellent effect is obtained. It is better to start injection from KI_2 and PC_5. When the patient's symptom disappeared, treatment can be discontinued thereafter. For the prolongation of the effect, it is very useful to put thumbtack needle at every point. Only by putting thumbtack needle (without any other acupuncture), excellent effect is often obtained.

§ 4 Chronic Urticaria (cf. p196)

Acute urticaria is fairly easy to cure by acupuncture treatment of LUNG Meridian (mainly U_7). There acupoint injection &/or thumbtack needle is mainly used. In most cases, itch sensation disappears rapidly after the injection, and sometimes exanthema reduces or disappears. As it is closely related with allergy, KI_2 and PC_5 is used together, and the effect seems better.

Treatment of chronic urticaria is not so easy. Itching decreases or disappears after the treatment, but exanthema hardly disappears. Adding treatment of KI_2 and PC_5 the effect seems to become somewhat better, and sometimes exanthema decreases. For the treatment of chronic urticaria, electro-acupuncture is better than acupoint injection. Method of treatment is almost the same as acute urticaria. Acupuncture may be useful as auxiliary method of Occidental Medicine and Kampo(Jp.) Medicine.

§ 5   Atopic Dermatitis

Main therapy for atopic dermatitis may be Occidental Medicine. Kampo(Jp.) medicine is sometimes very effective without side effects. But they are not always effective enough. Although acupuncture cannot play a leading role, it is sometimes very useful.

As mentioned before, one of the causes of disease progression is scratching due to itching. "To reduce itching" is very meaningful for "decrease scratching", and for this purpose, "treatment of LUNG Meridian (LU_7)" is often very effective.

Atopic dermatitis is regarded to have an aspect of autoimmune disease. So, point selection for the treatment of atopic dermatitis is LU_7, KI_2 and PC_5 regardless of the location of main lesion. Acupoint injection and intradermal- or thumbtack needle is useful enough for itching relief, but for the "treatment" of atopic dermatitis, electro-acupuncture is most useful.

Effect is not sure, but sometimes its effect is astonishing.

§ 6   Palmoplantar Pustulosis

Palmoplantar pustulosis is regarded as an intractable disease, but acupuncture therapy is often very effective.

This disease is autoimmune disease. So, basic point selection is KI_2 and PC_5. PERICARDIUM Meridian passes the palm, and KIDNEY Meridian passes the sole of the foot. Both points are on the meridians that pass the place of the lesion. Basic meridian selection for skin disease is LUNG Meridian ("Skin and hair belong to LUNG"). So, points for the treatment of palmoplantar pustulosis is LU_7, PC_5 and KI_2. Any methods of acupuncture are useful. For acupoint injection Vitamin B_{12} is mostly used because it is called "Vitamin of the nerve". .

Appearance of the effect is fairly rapid. Itch sensation usually disappears just after the treatment. The lesion becomes cleaner in a few days. Sometimes skin becomes almost normal. Duration of the effect varies. Most of patients are satisfied with the effect, and stop visiting in the course of treatment. So, final effect is mostly not clear. I confirmed only one case that showed complete recovery, but this method is surely effective and useful.

214 PART 6 PRACTICE OF ACUPUNCTURE

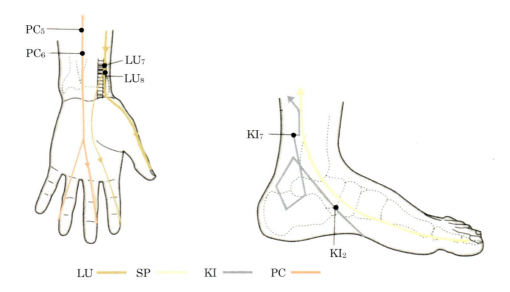

Fig.117 Points for Treatment of Palmoplantar Pustulosis

§ 7 IgA Nephropathy

IgA nephropathy is one of the progressive glomerulonephritis and it is regarded to be an autoimmune disease. Tonsillectomy and steroid pulse therapy is the usual therapeutic method of Occidental Medicine. But sometimes it is not effective enough.

There is an impressive case. It is only one case, but the case seems to indicate that acupuncture can be expected as a method of treatment of IgA nephropathy.

Patient was a male, 28 y. o. at initial visit. IgA nephropathy was found at 19 y. o. The preceding year of the first visit, he was diagnosed by biopsy of kidney as IgA nephropathy, in a group of relatively poor prognosis. He received tonsillectomy and steroid pulse therapy. But its effect was insufficient and urinary protein and urine occult blood reaction was continuously over 3+.

He had a slight fatigue, back pain and heavy shoulder stiffness, but otherwise he had no remarkable symptom. Pulse showed deficiency at all meridians (by the pulse diagnosis at 6 definite points).

At the initial visit, thumbtack needle (0.6mm) was tried putting on KI_2, PC_5 and BL_{64}. The reason to use BL_{64} is according to my impression about BLADDER, that its function seems to have urinary secretion.

After four days, the patient visited doctor in charge. The doctor was astonished as his urinary protein showed ±. Thereafter treatment of electro-acupuncture to KI_2,

PC5 and BL64, being added thumbtack needle on the same points after electro-acupuncture treatment, principally once a week.

After 11 days from the start of acupuncture, casual urinary protein decreased from 300 ~ 500mg/dl to 30mg/dl. After 3 weeks from the start of acupuncture, urinary occult blood showed negative. Subjective complaints soon disappeared completely.

Morning urinary protein evidently decreased after 5 weeks, and it shows almost always ±, sometimes + and sometimes negative. Urinary occult blood became almost always negative after 2yeas and 9months, and for these about 10 years it stayed negative.

This treatment is continuing mearly 13 years (at the period of 2019). Medication of steroid hormone is stopped over 10 years ago, and everything is going well.

This is only one case report. But this patient was aggressively treated by Occidental Medicine for 4 months, and high grade urinary protein and occult bleeding was not suppressed. In consideration of the effect of thumbtack needle (0.6mm) one time, and showing excellent effect of electro-acupuncture and thumbtack needle for over 10 years without steroid hormone, it could be estimated that acupuncture is effective for IgA nephropathy.

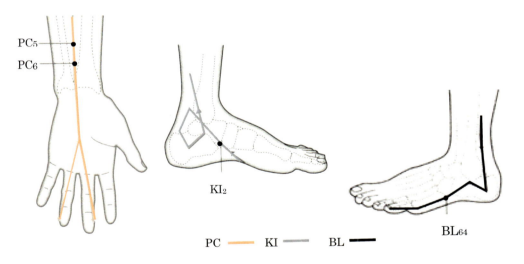

Fig.118   Points for IgA Nephropathy

216   PART 6 PRACTICE OF ACUPUNCTURE

§ 8 Myasthenia Gravis

Myasthenia gravis is an autoimmune disease, and it is yet intractable in spite of the development of investigation and methods of treatment. Thymus is closely related with this disease, and thymectomy is often very effective.

As mentioned before, PERICARDIUM must be thymus, and treatment of myasthenia gravis (ocular myasthenia) was tried using PC_5 and LR_3. Effect was unexpectedly good, and diplopia disappeared promptly.

Basic point selection is KI_2 and PC_5 (or PC_6), and points on the meridian that passes through the place of the aimed organ or muscle as Table 7.

Table 7 Meridians & Points for Myasthenia Gravis

Aimed Organ or Muscle	Meridian	Point
Basic Point	PC Merid.	PC_5 or PC_6 Kyoukei GB_{43}
	KI Merid.	KI_2
Symptom of Eye	LR Merid.	LR_3
	Auricle	Eye Point to Eye_2
M. Levator Palpebrae	TE Merid.	TE_3 (or TE_2)
	GB Merid.	GB_{41} or GB_{43}
	LR Merid.	LR_3
Adynamic Muscle	Corresponding Points Same as Selection for Pain	

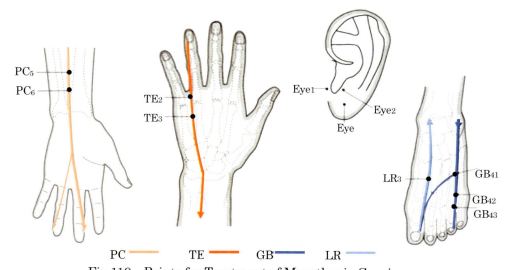

Fig.119 Points for Treatment of Myasthenia Gravis

Consequence of my experience (although number of cases is yet very small) is as described below.
1. Acupuncture therapy is effective for eyelid ptosis. Just after the treatment, patients were able to easily open the eye in all cases. In some cases, ptosis recovered completely. Duration of effect was half day to several days.
2. Acupuncture therapy is effective for diplopia, but effect is not sure.
   In some cases, diplopia disappeared just after the treatment, and in other case several times' treatments were necessary until the appearance of the effect. In one case, diplopia retrogressed temporally after treatment. No case of deterioration by acupuncture was experienced.
3. No effective case of muscle weakness was experienced.

§ 9   Sjögren's Syndrome

Sjögren's syndrome is an intractable disease, Even by Occidental Medicine, treatment is no better than palliative therapy. "Cure by acupuncture" will be impossible, but it is useful for treatment of some complaints.

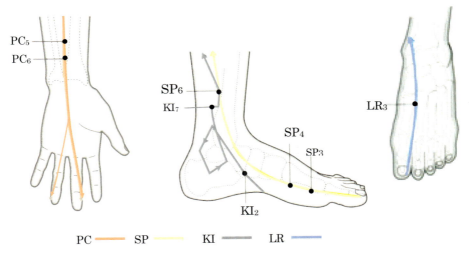

Fig.120 Points for Treatment of Sjögren's Syndrome

Sjögren's syndrome is autoimmune disease. The severest symptom for the patient is dehydrated feeling of the eye and the mouth. LIVER Meridian (LR) passes through the eye and inside of the cheek, SPLEEN Meridian (SP) spreads under the tongue and KIDNEY Meridian (KI) reaches the root of the tongue. So, points for treatment are PC$_5$, KI$_2$, SP$_4$ and LR$_3$.

The effect is good for all cases. Patients feel moist at the eye and in the mouth, just after the treatment. Long term effects are not yet clear.

§ 10 Fibromyalgia

The main symptom of fibromyalgia is pain. Treatment of pain is a favorite field of acupuncture. But effects of acupuncture are inferior compared with other pain. Acupoint injection with opiates or Pentazocine can sedate almost all kinds of pain. But I have no chance to try it for fibromyalgia.

Cause of fibromyalgia is not yet clear. Autoimmunity is regarded to be one of the causes. So, the treatment is tried adding KI_2 and PC_5 together with usual method of pain sedation. Effect seemed better than usual method of pain sedating acupuncture. But it is not yet sure.

§ 11 Alopecia Areata

Alopecia areata is regarded to be autoimmune disease, and steroid hormone is used for the treatment. Usually it happens at the head where GALLBLADDER Meridian (GB) (sometimes + BLADDER MERIDIAN) passes. So, point selection for treatment is KI_2, PC_5, GB_{41}, GB_{42} or GB_{43} (+BL_{64}) and LU_7 (because classic literature says "skin & hair belong to LUNG"). It must be noticed that many patients of this disease heals spontaneously. So, the effect should be judged carefully.

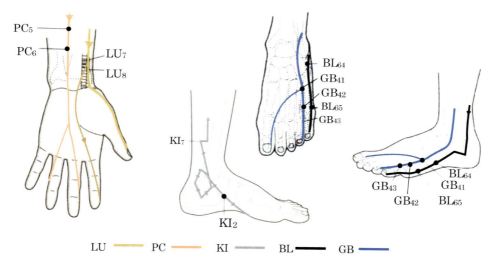

Fig.121 Points for Treatment of Alopecia Areata

There is one case of successful treatment. The patient had alopecia about 3cm in diameter which lasted over half a year, not changing its diameter, and Occidental therapy was not effective. She was given electro-acupuncture at KI_2, PC_5 and GB_{43}, and thereafter thumbtack needle was put for one week at the same points and LU_7.

After one month of this treatment, the part of alopecia was covered with short hair completely.

The process could not be observed exactly, but its progress seems to suggest that acupuncture could be one method of treatment of alopecia areata.

INDEX

A

abbreviation x
abdomen 154
   around navel 155
   epigastrium 155
   hypochondrium 155
   inguinal region 155
   lower abdomen 155
Acupoint Injection v, 8, 103, **121**
acupoint **12, 44**
acupuncture anesthesia 166
acupuncture needle 9
acupuncture point 12
allergic disease 209
Alopecia Areata 218
anesthesiology 165
anus 158
apparent paralysis 179
arm 151
Arm-SanriLI$_{10}$ 49
around shoulder joint 149
articular pain 172
artificial anus (erosion) 196
asthma-like symptom 191
Atopic Dermatitis **199**, 213
Attention
   after acupuncture therapy 104
   auricle 81
   deviation of points 49, 50, 60
   moxa needle 118
   obesity 187
Auricular Acupunture **119, 187**
autoimmune disease 209
auscultation 106

B

Back pain 156, **171**
balance 110
B-cun 46, 83
belong 16
Bladder 78
BLADDER Meridin (BL) 25

points 55
bleeding 126
blood letting 102
body acupuncture 5, 109, 115
bone proportion SUN(CUN) 46, **83**
bronchial asthma **190, 210**
Burning Mountain Method **100**

C

cancer pain 163
central nervous system 174
Cervico-brachial Syndrome 171
chest (anterior-&-lateral part) 152
chin (sknk) **70, 71**
ChoueGB$_2$ 60
Chronic urticaeia 212
ChuushoTE$_3$ **60**
classic meridian viii, 15,
compression fracture vertebra 167
connect 12, 16
CONCEPTION VESSEL (CV) 41
   point 63
contamination 128
contraindication 133
complication 126
constipation 186
copper-man 44

D

DaishouKI$_4$ 57
DaitsuiGV$_{14}$ 62
DairyouPC$_7$ 58
DEFICIENCY 1, 64, **68**
dehydrated feeling (mouth) 186
demerits
   aupuncture 3
   intradermal needle 96
   Thumbtack needle 96
   SSP 121
diabetic neuralgia 179
Diagnosis at 6 definite points **70**
digestive organ 185
diplopia 207
disinfection 89
dizziness 203

INDEX

depressive state 184
dysmenorrhea 192
menopausal disorder 193
dysuria 208

E

ear 201
easiest acupuncture v
effect
    appearance 124
    course 125
EkimonTE$_2$ 59
elbow joint 152
electro-acupuncture 102, **109**
emesis 193
epigastrium 155
estimation of pulse **73**
EXCESS 1, 64, **68**
EXTERIOR 64
extra meridian 13
eye (pain etc.) 207
eyelid acupuncture 120, **182**

F

face and mouth
    around the nose 144
    eye 139
    forehead 145
    lower jaw 142
    oral cavity and tongue 141
    throat 141
    toothache 140
    upper jaw / zygomatic area 143
Fibromyalgia 218
filiform needle 9, 109
    management 89
finger 152
Finger Pressure 123
FIVE ELEMENTS 78
Five Evils 79
Five Masters 79
Five Roots 79
Five Strangeness 79
flow of meridian 14,
foot 163

Foot-RinkyuuGB$_{41}$ 61
Fourteen Meridians 15
Frequency
    Acupuncture therapy 103
Front Position 70
fresh injury 167
Fu (float) **70, 71**
FukuryuuKI$_7$ 57
FuyouBL$_{59}$ 56

G

GaikanTE$_5$ 60
GALLBLADDER Meridian (GB) 34
    points 60
geizui 92
GekanST$_7$ 51
GekimonPC$_4$ 58
general rule of treatment
    allergic disease 209
    autoimmune disease 209
    dermal disease 195
    ophthalmology 206
    pain / stiffness / numbness 134
general chart vii
general meridian vii
genital region 158
Getting KI(QI) 84, 93, **94**
glaring all directions points 176
gluteal region 158
GokeiSI$_3$ 54
goushin 9
GoukokuLI$_4$ 49
GoshoBL$_5$ 55
GOVERNOR VESSEL (GV) 39
    Points 62
guide tube 89
Gynecology 192

H

hand 151
hand joint 152
head (except face) 135
    around center line 136
    outerside of center line ~ parietal 136
    temporal~retro-auricular region 137

    lateral forehead   137
    broad area / obscure region   137
hearing & smelling   65
hearing loss   201
HEART Meridian (HT)   22
    point   53
Herpes Zoster (fresh)   125, **197**
Hibiki (Getting KI(QI)   84, 93, **94**
hiccup   185
hip joint   161
Hirata's Twelve Reaction Zone   81
ho   66
How to operate "Tokki"   112
hypochondrium   155
HiyouBL58   55
HyakueGV20   63

I

IgA Nephropathy   214
impotence   22, 169, 208
IN   13, 64
infection   127
IngekiHT6   53
Inguinal region   155
InkokuKI10   57
indication
    acupuncture   5
INTERIOR   64
inspection   106
intercostal neuralgia   176
intersection   52, 58, 60
intradermal needle   10, **94**, 119

J

JigoeGB42   61

K

Kan   70
Kanjou   70
KankokuST43   51
KanshiPC5   58
KeikotsuBL64   56
KeikyoLU8   48
KekkaiSP10   52
KETSU(BLOOD)   1, 64

KI(QI)   1, 64
KIDNEY   77, 78, 209
KIDNEY Meridian (KI)   28
   Point **56**
knee joint   162
KonronBL60   56
KoukanLR2   61
KoukeiSI3   54
KoumyouGB37   60
KousaiLU6   48
KousonSP4   52
KyokuchiLU11   50
KyokusaBL4   55
KyokusenLR8   62
KyokutakuPC3   58
KyoukeiGB43   61
KyuukyoGB40   60

L

LARGE INTESTINE Meridian (LI)   **17**
  point   49
leaving needle   126
leg   160
Leg-SamriST36   45, 51
Liver Meridian (LR)   **37**,
    points   61
lower extremity
   foot   163
   hip joint   161
   knee joint   162
   leg   160
lower abdomen   155
LUNG Meridian (LU)   15
    point   48
Points of each meridian   47
Lumber pain   156, **171**

M

magnetic grain   123
malignant tumor   163
management of needle   86
manipulation   7, 99, 115
medical examination   64
meridian   12
meridian phenomenon   12

meridian point injection 103
meridian selection 107
   Organ and organ &/or tissue 76
   Resemblance of Organ and organ 77
   WATER Poisoning 77
   Five Element theory 78
merit
   acupuncture 2
   acupoint injection 103
   intradermal needle 95
   round skin needle 96
metabolic disease 185
methods of acupuncture 5
Middle Position 70
Morning sickness 193
motor paralysis **179, 182**
   facial nerve paralysis 179
   recurrent nerve Paralysis 181
   extremity 182
moxa needle 99, **115**
Myasthenia Gravis 216

N

NaikanPC$_6$ **58**
name of points 45
NaiteiST$_{44}$ 51
nausea 185
navel 155
neck 146
   back 146
   anterior &/or lateral part 147
needle 9
   insertion 89
   management 86
needle breakage 127
NenkokuKI$_2$ 57
Neuralgia 174
   Intercostal Neuralgia 176
   Post-herpetic Neuralgia (PHN) 176
   Sciatica 176
   Trigeminal Neuralgia 174
   diabetic neuralgia 179
nose 203

O

Obesty 187
observation 65
ocular hypertension 207
olfaction 106
OnryuuLI$_7$ 49
organ viii
orthopedics 165
oukotsuKI$_{11}$ 28
out of indication
   disease 131
      Electro-acupuncture 132
      Thumbtack Needle 132

P

pain 134
painless delivery 194
Palmoplantar Pustulosis 213
palpation 66, 107
   abdomen 66
   meridian 67
Penetrating Heaven Cooling method 101
PERICADIUM 78, 209
PERICARDIUM Meridian (PC) 31
   points **58**
pharmaco-acupuncture 103, 122
pharyngo-laryngeal region 204
point 12, **45**
   auricle 81
point injection 103, 122
point search 83
point selection **80**, 108
point taking 108
pollinosis 204, **210**
post-herpetic neuralgia 134, **176**
post-operative intestinal paresis 165
Postoperative pain 165
preliminary massage 89
premedication 165
principle
   acupuncture 1
   acupuncture therapy 6
   meridian selection 75
   point selection 80
process

    effect of acupuncture   124
    fresh Herpes Zoster   198
    needle insertion   89
    treatment of obesity   188
    whiplash syndrome   170
psychosis   184
pulse
    examination   72
    recording   73
pulse diagnosis   67, **70**
pulse examination   72

Q
questioning   66, 106

R
Rear Position   70
recurrent nerve paralysis   181
rebound   125, 177, 198
refractory fistula   168
ReidouHT$_4$ 53
ReikouLR$_5$ 62
RekketsuLU$_7$ 48
Retaining needle   **98,** 115
Round skin needle   11, **95,** 99, 79, 119, 188
ryoudouraku   83
RyoukyuuST$_{34}$ **51,** 185

S
sacral region   158
SanchikuBL$_2$ 55
SanganLI$_3$ 49
Saninkou SP$_6$ **52**
SanyourakuTE$_8$ 60
sensory paralysis   134, 179
sha   68
Shaku   70
Shakuchuu   70
shakudohou   46, 83
ShakutakuaLU$_5$ 48
Shikitaihyou   79
ShikouTE$_6$ 60
ShinmonHT$_7$ 53
SHOU   64
shoulder / shoulder joint   148

Spinal Canal Stenosis   172
Sjögren Syndrome   217
side effect   126, **130**
silver grain   123
ShoukaiHT$_3$ 53
ShoukaiSI$_6$ 54
ShoukaiKI$_5$ 57
ShoukouBL$_6$ 55
ShouzanBL$_{57}$ 55
skin cutting   89
skin penetration   92
    training   93
    without needle   91
SPLEEN   78
SMALL INTESTINE Meridian('SI)   24
    Points   54
smelling   65
SokkotsuBL$_{65}$ 56
somatoform disorder   184
SPLEEN Meridian (SP)   20
    points   52
SSP   84, 121
stimulation   6
balance   110
    strength   109
    time   109
    frequency (Herz)   109
STOMACH Meridian (ST)   18
    points   51
SUI(WATER)   64
SuisenKI$_6$ 58
Sun   70
Sunkou   70
Supplementation   1, **68, 97**
Surgery   165

T
TaienLU$_9$ 48
TaihakuSP$_3$ 52
TaishiouLR$_3$ 62
TaikeiKI$_3$ 57
TaimyakuGB$_{26}$ 60
TenseiTE$_{10}$ 59
TentotsuCV$_{22}$ 63
Thoracic Outlet Syndrime   171

throat   141
Thumbtack Needle   11, 95, 99
Tinnitus   202
Tokki (Getting Ki(Qi)   84, **94**
Tokki (instrument)   105, **111**
   control of stimulation   113
   trouble   114
TRIPLE ENERGIZER Meridian   32
   points   59
training of management of needle   89, 93
trsubo   44
TsuuriHT$_4$ 53
TsuutenBL$_7$ 55

U
urticarial   196
urolithiasis   208

V
vertebral fracture   167
vomiting   185

W
WankotsuSI$_4$ 54
Water   iii, 64, 77
Water acupuncture   103, 122
Well-Pass Route   83
whiplash syndrome   168

X

Y
YANG   13, 64
YIN   13, 64
YO-U   13, 64
YouchiTE$_4$ 59
YoukeiLI$_5$ 49
YoukouGB$_{35}$ 60
YoukokuSI$_5$ 54
YourouSI$_6$ 54
YousenKI$_1$ 56

Z
zou-fu   viii

Author's Biography

Author   Family Name : WATANABE   Given Name : Hiroshi
Address : 3-11-32, Chuo, Kofu-City, Yamanashi Pref., JAPAN
　　　　　Postal Code : 400-0032, Japan
　　　　　Tel : +81-55-233-7223
　　　　　e-mail : watnbeh@ybb.ne.jp
Date of Birth : 1926, Jan.29
Author's Affiliation : Yumura Spa Hospital

Academic background

1951	Bachelor of Medicine, University of Tokyo
1951	Internship at University of Tokyo
1960	Ph. D., University of Tokyo

Professional background

1952	Member of the 2nd Faculty of Surgery of Tokyo University
1961-65	Chair, Dep. of Surgery at Kokuho Asahi Chuo Hospital
1968-70	Chair, Dep. of Surgery at Moro Hospital
1970-82	Chair, Dep. Surgery at Yamanashi Prefectural Central Hospital
1982-87	Chair of the Board and Director at Ichinomiya Spa Hospital
1988-93	Chair, Dep. of Surgery at Isawa Spa Hospital
1993-95	Vice-director at Ryuo Surgical Hospital
1996-2002	Vice-director at Kyosai Central Clinic
2002-05	Chair, Dep. of Oriental Medicine at Shirane Tokushukai Hospital
2005-12	Director at Fujien Nursing Home
2012-17	Director at Tamaho Care Center Nursing Home
2018	Member of Yumura Spa Hospital

Teaching profession

1974-98	Docent at Department of Education, University of Yamanashi
1979-92	Docent of Surgery II, Yamanashi Medical University

Experiences regarding Oriental Medicine

1973-78	Studied acupuncture under Dr. MANAKA Yoshio & Dr.TANI Michio at Japanese Association of Eastern Medicine.

1984-86	Chair, Yamanashi district, Councilor at Japan Society of Acupuncture and Moxibustion (JSAM)
1986-2000	Board member at JSAM
1990	Certified as Kampo medical specialist by the Japan Society for Oriental Medicine
1999	Certified as academic specialist by JSAM
2000-04	Auditor at JSAM
2001	Advisor of Financial group of Buenos Aires Society of Anesthesiologists
2004	Medical instructor of Kampo Medicine authorized by the Japan Society for Oriental Medicine.

Published books (in Japanese)

·Hari wo shiranakutemo dekiru tsubo chusha chiryo
(Acupoint Injection for Those not Familiar with Acupuncture) from Kimpodo, 1996, revised edition 2002
·Ika no tameno wakariyasui hari-chiryo
(Intelligible Acupuncture Treatment for Doctors) from Kimpodo 2001

Easy Method of ACUPUNCTURE
Based on Meridian Theory

Copyright ©2019 by WATANABE Hiroshi All rights reserved.

No part of this publication may be reproduced, stored in a retrieval system, or transmitted in any form or by any means, electronic, mechanical, photocopying, recording, or otherwise, without the prior permission of the publisher.

Published in Japan.   ISBN978-4-86584-356-9

For information contact : BookWay
ONO KOUSOKU INSATSU CO.,LTD.
62, HIRANO-MACHI, HIMEJI-CITY, HYOGO 670-0933 JAPAN
(Phone) 079-222-5372 (Fax) 079-244-1482